Pamela Armstrong is a broadcaster and journalist, she has worked in both hard news and current affairs as well as general interest programmes.

After fronting ITN's flagship 'News at Ten', she presented a variety of programmes for the BBC including 'The Pamela Armstrong Show', 'Daytime Live' and 'Breakfast Time'. She has anchored for BBC World Service Television and presented the ground-breaking health series, 'Well-Being' on Channel 4 where its popular appeal took it to the top of the ratings.

She lives in London and is heading towards menopause.

Jacky Fleming is a best-selling cartoonist. Her books, *Be a Bloody Train Driver*, *Never Give Up* and *Falling in Love* are published by Penguin.

THE PRIME OF YOUR LIFE

Self help during Menopause

Pamela Armstrong

HEADLINE

First published in 1994
by HEADLINE BOOK PUBLISHING

10 9 8 7 6 5 4 3 2 1

ISBN 0 7472 4438 3

Typeset by
Letterpart Limited, Reigate, Surrey

Printed and bound in Great Britain by
HarperCollins Manufacturing, Glasgow

HEADLINE BOOK PUBLISHING
A division of Hodder Headline PLC
Headline House
79 Great Titchfield Street
London W1P 7FN

For all the women who have
contributed to this book

Contents

Introduction

This is a book that doesn't need to be read in sequence.

It's a book to be dipped into. Head for the sections that answer your current questions. The chapter on sex, for example, comes about halfway through. There's also a large section on self-help, including food, exercise and complementary medicines.

It is designed for everyone – especially the 50 per cent or so of women who don't use HRT.

Many women happily take HRT and it brings relief. The self-help chapters will interest those on HRT who want to experiment with recipes and remedies which will work alongside their medical treatment.

They're also there for the women who don't need to take HRT, or those who can't even start because of their medical history. Some find on trying HRT that it simply doesn't work for them; others want to go the natural route.

The first part of the book is a quick rundown of what the menopause is – how our bodies function and what may happen during those inevitable hormonal changes.

If you're considering taking HRT you might like to explore the different areas of debate. And if you do decide to use it, it may be worth looking at the chapter on you and your GP so that you can work out sooner, rather than later, how you'd like to manage your own treatment.

It's always worth keeping a weather eye on the latest gen. New information is emerging thick and fast and there may be just one nugget in there that could make a big difference for you.

The menopause has had a mixed press. For some women

1

it's the best thing that's happened to them for many a year. For others it's a time of physical upheaval and mental adjustment.

All some women want is confirmation that it's happening, and that it's natural. Others decide to treat their symptoms either with HRT or complementary medicines. A recent newspaper survey showed that nine out of ten people have used complementary medicine at one time or other, so it's gaining popularity all the time.

A number of therapies are explored. It's certainly not a definitive list and there's room to investigate any others that might help. For instance I've come across an old recipe which used to be a remedy for hot flushes and consists of one and a half pints of vintage clear London porter, or a glass of Rhenish wine. If anyone can find the ingredients, let alone try them, I'd be delighted to hear if it works . . .

The important thing with the menopause seems to be to junk as many of the myths about it as we can.

The menopause does not make you shoplift. It does not make you mad. It does not turn you into an alcoholic. It does not make you old, and bald, and withered. Other things in life might. But not the menopause.

It's worth remembering that a lot of what is written about 'the change' is written by doctors, or will certainly be informed by what they have to say. They write responsibly and with knowledge. But they are specialists in a narrow field, dealing almost solely with problems. Inevitably they write from the perspective of people who, on the whole, see the more difficult aspects of the situation most of the time.

The menopause can be uncomfortable for some women. But for many others it is not a problem, just a normal physical process. It has varying effects that, though irritating, never rise above being manageable. It's important to remain resistant to scare stories. Do not let anyone define your menopause for you. Trust your instincts. If you need help seek it. And be aware of the many options available to you, from your GP to the local nutritionist. If you want to ride it out, do so. It's an entirely natural process. It will pass. Don't be railroaded into thinking anything else.

The menopause is a threshold. The whole of the rest of your life beckons. Good luck.

CHAPTER 1

The word is . . .

'Most of us don't want to be glamour queens and have sixteen toy boys before breakfast. We just want to get back to normal. Women come here in despair and think they're going mad. "I thought nobody had that," they say. "I didn't even know it was a symptom. I thought I was the only one." There is amazement and relief when they hear that other women go through the same things. And they think it's a miracle what we can do for them.'
Doctor at a Well Woman clinic.

'You get a sore throat treated. That's taken seriously. Why in hell shouldn't you get your sore, dry vagina treated too?'
The same doctor.

'It's disturbing because you worry about what to do all the time. I don't want to put drugs in my system. But I don't have that much confidence in nature either. Evolution doesn't always work for the best.'
Sasha, forty-four.

'In some ways my generation's lucky. We've sort of always been fashionable. And Germaine Greer's making sure it's staying that way now she's banging the drum about the menopause. Menopause is coming out of the closet.'
Terry, forty-seven.

'It's hard to know if it was the menopause beginning. I definitely had a serious depression. But my husband was out

of work at the same time. So it could have been that. How can you tell?'
Barbara, forty-three.

'I want to be able to chat about it like we do about periods, and childbirth. I resent that I can't talk openly about it.'
Cal, forty-five.

'I've taken a lot of pregnancy tests lately. Oh my God, I think. The menopause or pregnancy? Which is worse?'
Bel, forty-four.

'I thought I was having my first hot flush. But I'd left the electric blanket on.'
Jan, forty-four.

'I was devastated in many respects. I'm not married, never have been married. And I'd make a good mother. I know I would. I found it hard. Some of my women friends with kids complain about having the drag of periods and all those menstrual hassles. And I think, hang on a minute. At least you've got kids at the end to show for it. But I don't. And it's tough.'
Kath, forty-four.

'Some women regard the only sign of menopause as having wonky periods. But there's one woman I know with regular periods who's been irritable and difficult and bad tempered, and she doesn't put it down to hormonal swings. "Oh, I haven't any signs of it at all," she chirps. And I think, you don't know what an absolute sod you've been for the last six years.'
Liz, forty-seven.

'The thing about hot flushes, when you get them a lot, is it unbalances you. You've just got comfortable, reading a book, watching the telly and someone says something that excites you. Or the doorbell rings and you rush for it. And you begin

to recognise that it is the sudden movement or change that brings them on. There's sudden upheaval and you go from relative comfort to discomfort. It makes you stop wanting to do things. Or to stop wanting to do them so fast. It slows you down. And that's irritating. It cramps your style.'
Elsa, forty-seven.

'I think a lot of women carry on taking HRT when they don't need it. They like the cycle. They like the monthly period. It makes them still think they're "women" in some way.'
Bea, forty-eight.

'Some patients come to me and I diagnose them as menopausal. And they react like I've said a dirty word. "Oh, no!" they say, "That's not what it is at *all*." '
Homeopathist.

'It's almost as if nature has designed a way to make old ladies. I like that. We need them. They're valuable in some way to society. Maybe the eighteen and nineteen-year-olds who're dropping babies left, right and centre need their grannies. Someone has to pass on the information of how to do it . . . Menopause is essential. I don't want to go on being fertile till I'm old. In the olden days women didn't grow old. They died relatively young. They had their fifteen children. And it killed them. These days we're all much healthier and keep on going for ages. Imagine being pregnant at *seventy-five*, and dying of *that* then.'
Judith, forty-seven.

CHAPTER 2

Will I grow a moustache?

It's not such a crazy question. For many women who don't know any better, the whole idea of the menopause is one they'd rather put on the back burner – permanently. It's shrouded in ignorance and fear. Isn't it that time of life when older women suddenly come over all peculiar? Isn't that the time when perfectly sane and well balanced citizens turn into screaming viragos? Haven't they been seen to prowl the streets at night shaking their fists at the moon and visibly sprouting facial hair?

This nonsense gets put about because the whole subject has been so taboo for so long. We all know that anything to do with women's sexuality has always been dealt with by half-truths and embarrassed murmurings.

That's changing. And not least because women have been getting feisty and demanding a better deal for themselves. And to its credit, the medical world has sat up and listened.

But even so, the result of years of shadows and silence is that many women suddenly find themselves at the beginning of the menopause, unsure and unknowing. There is a dread. They think it's a time when their breasts will atrophy, their vagina will shrink, sex will be over and so inevitably will life.

It's a pretty bleak image. It's frightening.

And it's wrong. Wrong. Wrong.

There is so much cultural clutter that confuses. First, let's not insult anyone's intelligence here by pretending all women sail through without difficulty. It can be uncomfortable. It can be distracting. It can be depressing. But over and above everything else it is *normal*. And it passes.

Our bodies are programmed for puberty, reproduction and

menopause from the moment we are conceived. But sometimes it takes a while for us to accept changes which are inevitable, particularly if we've got mixed feelings about them.

The negative attitudes we bring to the menopause often have less to do with its physical aspects than the mental ones. What concerns us are ingrained feelings about femininity, sexual appeal, self-image and ideas about social and personal worth – all of which may be thrown into question.

Life is tough enough for women when they're 'socially useful', having kids and working. How much tougher that can be made to seem when the vital ingredient of fertility is swept away.

Sure, not everyone wants kids. And even if they have them, the raising and nurturing of a family is, for most women, only one strand in lives that are multi-faceted and various. But even so, there is that notion that lurks at the back of the mind – once you're no longer capable of reproducing, it's time for the scrap heap.

It must come from some deep and primitive part of the brain. A part that deals only with physical survival. A part that developed in the ages before there was language and catastrophic population explosion.

It cuts deep and holds great power. For most women, feeling female is inextricably tied up with having a womb that works. When it doesn't, there can be confusion, loss and uncertainty.

Even if we know logically that women are more than a womb on two legs, emotionally it can be a different story.

It's complicated. With the menopause, body and mind are affected and that can carry over into the emotions, your family, your work, your whole life.

Just understanding what's going on helps. Many women sail through the menopause. Some don't. This book is for those who want to put in a bit of footwork, so that as the change in their bodies unfolds they are willing and able to let go of a past that is over, and turn to a future that can beckon with promise.

Some women find it the most liberating time of their lives. Isn't that ironic? I can remember in the early days of women's lib, it was the youngsters who thought they were revolutionising the world. And yet it was some of the older women who were going through the most profound changes. The youngsters still had an uncompromising twenty years of childbirth and child-rearing ahead of them. Whatever else they contributed, most of them were locked inexorably into that treadmill. How more biologically programmed can you get than that?

Some of the women who were truly freeing up their lives were the ones who were stepping off that treadmill. No longer being defined by their sexuality, no longer bound by social expectations and conventions, they were carving out a way of life that more genuinely reflected their inner needs and wants. That's real freedom.

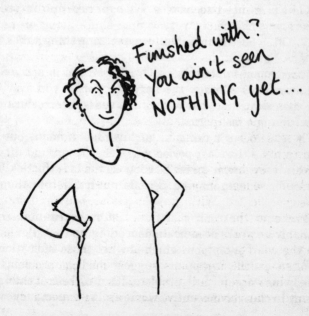

Finished with? You ain't seen NOTHING yet...

CHAPTER 3

What exactly are we talking about here?

Is the menopause a joke, a medical condition, or a crisis? From the disinformation that's been put about over the years, you'd be excused for thinking it's any of those.

There's nothing like knowing what you're talking about to help you feel more confident about the way you are going to choose to manage your menopause. It's useful when you go to your GP with perhaps those first early twinges and doubts, to have a broad grasp of the issues that need to be raised.

There's no need to have a PhD in medicine in order to understand the really very simple shifts going on in your body. Often just being able to name something takes away the anxiety.

'*Mens*' means monthly in Greek. '*Pause*' is self evident. '*Menopause*' is actually the very last period you ever have. The menopause is what we call the years before, during and after that one last period.

There's no such thing as an average woman, but most women have that last period when they're around fifty. For some, a very few, it comes as early as the late thirties. There are other women having periods naturally into their late fifties.

Whatever the timing of that last menstruation, there'll probably be years of indications leading up to it. I'm loath to use the word symptoms which is what those indications are so often called. Symptoms suggest medical problems. The menopause needn't be a problem. It's a process of change.

Until relatively recently, women's life expectancy was so

much lower. Many died before they even got to menopause, the rest during or just after. In Roman times the average lifespan for a woman was twenty-nine years. Even by 1841, in England and Wales it had gone up to only forty-two. But by 1970 it was seventy-five, an increase of sixty-eight per cent during the last century. Now many of us can expect to live one whole third of our lives after it's over.

In fact, these 'new' women are pioneers. There have never been so many women completely freed from fertility for so long. The birth rate is falling in the First World and the real number of older people increasing. One in ten people today are over sixty. By 2030 it'll be one in six.

In America by the year 2010, forty million women will be going through or past their menopause. TV's 'The Golden Girls' are only the tip of the iceberg. Imagine the political power of a pressure group that large. For too long, older women have been made invisible, but time and numbers are on their side.

By the by, apparently women in America have far more fear of the menopause than women in Europe. American society is so youth-oriented that anything that suggests so much as a whisper of ageing or change gives many of them the screaming abdabs.

So much of the anxiety about the menopause has to do with fear of ageing. One minute you're juicy and vibrant and full of energy, and the next you're a wizened old crone, bent over with a dowager's hump. It doesn't work quite like that. Some women's menopause can take up to ten years. For others it's four to five. And for a few it seems to happen overnight. For many it is gradual and slow, and so are its effects.

But nevertheless in a culture which worships youth, you're going to get your comedians like Joan Rivers telling jokes about the dimple in her chin really being her navel – it's just that she's had so many facelifts. She knows her audience. There's a chilling ring of despair wrapped up in the laughs which cracks like that generate.

In Europe there seems to be a more forgiving attitude to

ageing, and that can make the whole thing easier. Much is clearly in the mind. And that's encouraging because there's a lot you can do about it.

Your body is programmed from the moment you are conceived to stop being fertile at a precise time in your life. It will be your time, and it will happen to you in your own unique way.

There are more post-menopausal women alive today than there have ever been before. Frankly, society is still writing the rule book on the subject. We're still drawing the map. Women like Joan Collins are rewriting history when it comes to attitudes to the older woman. But she's only one stereotype. Each one of us is going to bring something new to the table. The only way to be part of this huge tide of change is to get out there and carve it out for ourselves. Or someone else will do it for us. And we all know what that's done to women's lives in the past.

CHAPTER 4

Body clock

Let's get right back to square one. From the moment we're born, our bodies begin to gear up for our fertile years.

Each baby girl has a whacking two million egg-forming cells in her ovaries. It's just as well because many of those follicles, as they're called, are already dead and gone by the time puberty kicks off. By then, there are only around forty thousand left. And no new ones are ever produced.

Puberty usually begins in the early teens, when a few follicles ripen every month, triggered by the young girl's newly functioning hormones. A hormone is simply a natural chemical compound, made and released by a variety of glands around the body, creating automatic physical responses wherever it is sent.

The brain gives the order. The hormone carries the message. The targeted body part does what it's told. From the outside it looks as if we have an internal clock. From its rhythm comes the ebb and flow of all our body cycles.

In the old days doctors specialising in 'those funny female bits' used to consider their sphere of influence the area of the torso stretching from the waist to the top of the thighs. Which is why they misunderstood so much.

That's all changed. Not least since 1917 when a Dr Papanicolaou (of pap smear fame) noticed that vaginal cells altered depending on what time of the month it was. The hunt for the hormone was on. A real understanding of the sensitivity of the chemical ebb and flow began to emerge.

MISSION CONTROL

Way up in the bony cavity at the base of the brain nestles the pituitary gland. It's a small, round, pea-like piece of soft tissue. The pituitary releases a hormone called follicle-stimulating hormone. It quite literally tickles those egg-forming cells in the ovaries into action. When follicle-stimulating hormone is released, ten to twenty follicles begin to ripen.

Usually in a production you get one star of the show. Well, here we've got two. And they're a great double act. In this particular drama there are essential supporting artists like follicle-stimulating hormone who do the warm-ups. But then it's time for the first major player to take centre stage. And that's the hormone, oestrogen.

Once follicle-stimulating hormone has done the business and got the follicles going, the ovary swings into action.

The ovary isn't just a storehouse of potential eggs. It too is a gland in its own right. As the follicle develops, it begins to manufacture and secrete that first star of the show, oestrogen.

So at the beginning of the cycle, the levels of oestrogen in the blood begin to rise. And at first, ironically, that oestrogen begins to work as a block, to stop the pituitary gland producing any more of its follicle-stimulating hormone.

And so the ping-pong match begins. Each hormone tries to outdo the other in the amount that is produced.

For the pituitary gland, it's a bit like getting a fat smack. It gets stopped in its tracks. But it's a temporary block and it's called *negative* feedback. This negative feedback results in the pituitary briefly producing less follicle-stimulating hormone.

The ovaries continue to produce even more of *their* hormone, oestrogen. So the levels of oestrogen rise. As the oestrogen goes up, the pituitary in its turn suddenly goes into full steam ahead to compensate. This time it releases a new compound called luteinising hormone, plus some more follicle-stimulating hormone.

This return of serve is called *positive* feedback.

Confused? Imagine what it's doing to your body!

Somehow it all comes together in a precise crescendo, because after all that activity, the luteinising hormone does what it's meant to do – it triggers ovulation. An egg is released.

In the ovaries, the stimulated follicles vibrate in expectant anticipation. Each one has the potential to be the belle of the ball. But only one will be chosen.

The luteinising hormone is particularly clever. It will isolate the biggest and the best. In fact, that particular follicle will be visible to the naked eye. Luteinising hormone encourages the follicle, which will be blown up tight like a tiny balloon, to burst away from the ovary and make its journey to the womb via the Fallopian tubes.

So begins the survival of the fittest.

And that is ovulation. Simply the liberation of the ripened follicle from the ovary. The whole process has taken roughly fourteen days. It is around now that the oestrogen level peaks. And it's around now that women are fertile.

MEANWHILE

Back in the ovary, the empty follicle turns into what's called the corpus luteum, or yellow body, and that produces yet more of the hormone oestrogen, plus the other female hormone, progesterone.

Progesterone is the second star of the show, and we'll be getting to that in a moment.

First, let's look at what oestrogen gets up to in that first half of the menstrual cycle.

During those first fourteen days, the oestrogen works on building up the lining of the womb. In the second half of the cycle, the progesterone joins in. The lining grows thicker. This lining is called the endometrium and it resembles nothing so much as a sponge.

As well as helping the bulking up process, progesterone stimulates the lining of the womb to develop lots of tiny mucus glands which secrete a nutritious, succulent fluid in preparation for possible conception.

If there is no conception, the yellow body, or corpus luteum, dies. The oestrogen and progesterone levels fall right back. And the lining of the womb, the thickened spongy endometrium, falls away.

Part of the sponge-like function of the endometrium is to collect as much blood as possible to provide the healthiest environment for a baby. When the lining goes, the blood goes too, and we get a monthly bleeding – or period.

The time this usually takes is another fourteen days, hence the average twenty-eight-day spell between periods. But that's the average. Many women have completely normal cycles that can be longer, or shorter. The shortest ever recorded was all of eleven days. The longest cycle ever measured was one hundred and fifty days. But those last two are so rare, they practically fall off the graph.

So the average woman has a twenty-eight-day cycle – yet within her lifetime even that will change. When a young girl first starts her periods, her cycle will often be around thirty-five days. That cycle then gradually condenses during her life, until her early forties when it begins to expand again. The average cycle then is about fifty to fifty-two days.

And ovulation itself changes too. Although you started life with a couple of million of those egg-forming cells, by the early to mid-forties, they've reduced to around eight thousand – and only a few of those will ripen.

Women in the later stages of their fertile life produce more follicle-stimulating hormone from the pituitary gland than they did when they were younger. But even so, ovulation doesn't happen at every cycle and without it, no progesterone is made either. So overall, the production of progesterone and oestrogen begins to dwindle.

Menopause is beginning.

CHAPTER 5

Vicky's story

I just couldn't drum it into my GP's head that I was menopausal.

The problem was that I was having completely regular periods. If you ever have the misfortune to have a GP who only recognises irregular periods as the first and main symptom of menopause, I feel for you.

But it's a proven physical fact that women's bodies start deteriorating after thirty-five. I was in my early forties and I started having bodily changes I'd never experienced in my life before. I'm convinced it was the menopause starting. And he just wouldn't listen.

I felt I was suffering from PMS, not just before periods, but every day of the month. I was over-sensitive. I was on edge.

At work I'd suddenly lost all confidence. I'd been giving presentations for years and then all at once I started fumbling and getting nervous. There was a real dent in my self-image.

I went to my doctor who was on holiday, so I got one of the male GPs in the practice. One of those who barely look up from the prescription pad. He said I had water retention. And how common that was, and gave me pills.

Which didn't make a blind bit of difference because I then subsequently went to a homeopath who diagnosed hypoglycaemia – low blood sugar. Who's to say that isn't all part of the hormonal change for some women? I had the menopausal symptoms of irritability and loss of energy. They come from low blood sugar, but you listen to the number of menopausal women saying that's what they've got too. I was going

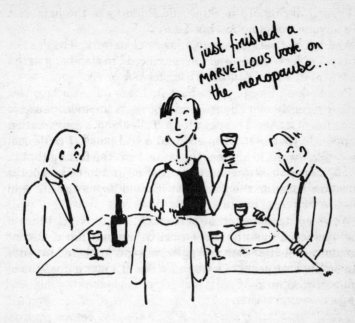

I just finished a MARVELLOUS book on the menopause...

through a change. How did that doctor know it wasn't *the* change?

Then I got this tiredness. Different from anything I've ever known. I could have just fallen asleep at the drop of a hat, any time of day, anywhere. My nerve endings in my jaws and my hands started to feel raw. I felt jangly all over. The doctor wondered if I needed a good holiday, or was over-stressed. I work for myself. I am successful. I have my own business. I'm beholden to no one. I'm solvent. I love my job. But I was *jangly*. I wasn't stressed – and he said take a good tonic.

So, back to the homeopath who diagnosed an allergy to coffee. Sudden negative reactions to foods and drinks you've been used to for years is definitely something that can happen in the menopause. I dropped the coffee and the 'jangly' feeling has gone. And another thing these days: I'd never eat a curry late at night. I wouldn't get to sleep. It's OK in the day. But my system just can't take it later on.

I've got drying of the skin. And thinning of the hair. Not so's anyone would notice, but I do.

And yet my periods are regular as clockwork. They're not heavy. I'm forty-seven and I'm convinced I'm slap-bang in the middle of it. And that I have been for five or six years.

People don't like to talk about it. I was out at a business dinner recently and I'd just read a book on the menopause so I was full of it. And I brought it up. Talk about a conversation stopper. It was as if I'd introduced a bad smell. I could feel they didn't want to address the issue. I got the feeling that to them, menopausal women were past it, and to talk about it somehow added to the possibility it could happen at all. And these were young women.

We've got to change that perception. I'm convinced that if one has good health and sufficient money for a decent standard of living, then the ages between forty and seventy can be the best years of a woman's life. It's just a question of being in good nick.

CHAPTER 6

The beginning of the end before the new beginning

What are the signs? When does 'It' begin? How will it feel? Are the scare stories true? It's called 'the change' for good reason. How is it going to change me?

The menopause is a voyage into the unknown. As that unknown approaches ever nearer, it's worth having a grasp of the broad issues and range of choices available. The newcomer, aware of the options, will have added confidence and extra knowledge. Both can help as you navigate one of life's major transitions.

So what should we expect? Life seems normal. The juices flow. Energy pulses round the body. And then, perhaps suddenly, or perhaps imperceptibly, the gears begin to change of their own accord. The machine isn't going from nought to sixty m.p.h. in ten seconds any more. In fact, some days you wonder whether you've got the energy to get out of bed at all.

WHAT IS GOING ON?

Something fundamental is changing. From deep inside your body a different tune is beginning to emerge. And like it or not, you're having to dance to its beat.

The indications of menopause are various. Some women's bodies will respond by throwing up one major symptom that cannot be ignored. Others may have a variety of mild signs that they can ride easily. One woman I know simply got engorged breasts, just before she had her (increasingly irregular) periods. Her remedy was to turn her body more gently so that her breasts didn't move too suddenly, and wear a bra in bed on the one or two nights when they were at their most tender. That was her menopause.

A lot of women think that they'll be able to work out when their menopause will start by back-tracking to when puberty started. The logic being if they started puberty early, then they'll start the menopause early too. And if their periods started later, then so too will their menopause.

Not so. It's tantalising, and for some women unnerving, not to know when the change is going to begin. But there is no way of telling. If you have a troubled gynaecological history it doesn't mean you'll have a bad menopause, and vice versa.

It's possible you may follow your mother's pattern. But apart from that, all you can do is carefully monitor your body. Watch for those changes and remain sensitive to the messages that it sends out. When it does begin, you'll know.

It's hardly likely you've got a path. lab tucked away in a corner of the kitchen, so you won't be able to monitor the hormonal shifts literally – just the effects.

But this broadly is what is going on.

STEPPING OUT OF TIME

From the age of about forty or so, all the hormones that we met recently begin to orchestrate themselves a little differently. Up till now they've happily engaged in their monthly symphony of cooperative collaboration. But the conductor begins to change the tempo and emphasis.

It's thought the cells in the ovaries, surrounding the waiting follicles, simply get less receptive to the hormones sent out by the pituitary gland. So the potential eggs aren't properly stimulated and don't get released. It's a bit like listening to someone saying the same thing over and over again. After a while you begin to tune out, and it can even lose its meaning.

But the body doesn't give up. It's aware of its poor response, so the pituitary tries to up the ante by secreting even more follicle-stimulating hormone. Anything to get those little bundles of human potential up and running.

As more follicle-stimulating hormone gets sent out, there's clearly more of it in the system. And this changes the proportions between follicle-stimulating hormone and luteinising hormone which is still being systematically released in the same amounts.

This means ovulation is less likely, and for some women periods become irregular.

Time passes. The ovaries change. The egg cells, or follicles, begin to disappear. Not only that, but the follicles' response to follicle-stimulating hormone lessens even more.

Yet again, the body's internal sense system rallies. Even more follicle-stimulating hormone is secreted, and again its level in the blood rises. The pituitary rallies heroically and as well as increasing levels of follicle-stimulating hormone, it now also increases production of luteinising hormone. So levels of that in the blood begin to rise too.

It's a valiant attempt, but eventually the egg cells either disappear, or they stop responding to the messages being sent out via both hormones from the pituitary gland.

Because of that, the level of oestrogen falls. No eggs are produced, so progesterone levels fall too as it was the follicles surrounding the eggs that used to make the progesterone.

The uterus is no longer stimulated.

Menstruation stops.

THE SHOCK OF THE NEW

In a way, menopause catapults us into withdrawal symptoms. For some women it's gradual. For others it feels like cold turkey. You've had the female sex hormones coursing through your body non-stop for thirty-five years or so; at the very least you'll be used to them, if not addicted.

When they stop, there's an adjustment to make.

Oestrogen and progesterone affect many areas of the body, not just the reproductive ones. We know they build up the lining of the womb. But they don't stop there. They're builders of body tissue, all over the body.

For instance, when puberty starts, you'll probably remember the change in and around your vulva. What was a flat slitlike surface plumps out. There's a growth of hair, the labia increase in size, as does the clitoris.

So too with the vagina. Oestrogen stimulates its lining, making it thicker and more pliable. That means it's easier for the penis to more safely deliver sperm.

We've heard how the double act of the female hormones work their minor miracle on the womb itself. Oestrogen first, then progesterone, coordinating during the twenty-eight-day cycle.

After the menopause, the loss of these two hormones will affect other areas of tissue as well – the skin, the skeleton, the heart and blood vessels, the blood, the urinary tract including the bladder, and the breasts.

BUT HANG ON A MINUTE

As I said, the levels of hormones do fall; indeed, are greatly reduced. But they don't disappear completely. The ovaries continue to secrete oestrogens for many years after the menopause. Just a lot, lot less.

After the menopause, levels of follicle-stimulating hormone and luteinising hormone actually increase. Oestrogen reduces but, via another route, does still continue to be produced in small doses elsewhere in the body.

Funnily enough, our bodies also produce the male hormone, testosterone, or androgen, also from the ovaries. This too reduces after the menopause, but not as much as the reduction in oestrogen. So, relatively, there is now more male hormone circulating. They say this may be the reason for the increased facial hair that appears on *some* menopausal women.

So the answer to the million dollar question, 'Will I grow a moustache?' is a very qualified 'perhaps'. But if you do, there are permanent remedies like electrolysis, which will quickly get rid of anything you want dealt with.

And it might help to remember that the higher levels of androgens can lessen some of the effects of menopause. On balance you're probably better off with them, than without.

SWINGS AND ROUNDABOUTS

The blood levels of both oestrogen and the androgens go up and down during the day, and have different levels on different days too.

But the reason for these swings still isn't known. So it's well nigh impossible to really fix on the fluctuations in any one woman's hormones as they're so individual and erratic. And that makes the linking of those internal shifts to the presenting symptoms of the menopause almost impossible too.

The hormonal mechanism is very subtle. It's such a sensitive mechanism. And it's different for every woman. And different at different times for the same woman.

It can be exasperating, but monitoring and treatment can still help.

CHAPTER 7

It's not all in the mind

I'm always reminded of the late Les Dawson when I think of the ways women's woes were swept under the carpet for years.

There was that woman he acted out who would always start her sentences, yet never finish them. Instead you'd get the beginning of an interesting titbit of gossip, always with some sexual innuendo. But it would be lost in a collapse of pursed lips, knowing, coy glances from under the eyelashes, tut-tuts and sighs.

'Well, I never! I've never known the likes of it before. Who'd have thought it! You know her up there, with the thingamummmy wrong with her whatsit. Mmmmmmmmmmm. Well . . .!!!!!!!!!!!!'

Well, *what*?

It's funny to watch these days. But it really was like that then. It's OK to see it parodied now, but can you imagine trying to communicate personal problems to a (very likely male) doctor in a sexual climate like that?

There must have been so much untold pain and discomfort. Women with very real and specific 'female trouble' would, if menopausal, be going to their doctors with hot flushes, dry vaginas and problematic periods. Not easy to describe when most things in that arena were dealt with by euphemisms, embarrassed fudging and half-truths. I bet more of them than would care to remember ended up talking about the pain in their big toe. If they went to the doctor at all.

Perhaps that's why there is so much dread today associated with the menopause. Sure, the underpinning anxiety surrounding the whole menopausal issue is mainly based on

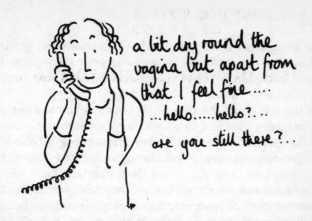

a bit dry round the vagina but apart from that I feel fine....
...hello.....hello?...
are you still there?...

fears about ageing. But putting that aside for a moment, I'm sure there's also a collective memory among women, simmering under the surface, which has very real experience of pain and discomfort. And it's a pain and discomfort that was probably easily treatable, if not avoidable.

There was so much more suffering than necessary because women did just put up with it in silence. In fact, a survey across Europe in the Seventies found British women in particular more stoic and more prepared to use the stiff upper lip to get them through. Indeed only 36 per cent of British women, the lowest number across the Continent, even knew there *was* any medical treatment at all. Residues of that rather spooky silence percolate through the generations even yet.

Yes, things are easier now because we have new drugs which weren't available then. And so much more is known. But it still doesn't explain the levels of fear and anxiety I've come across. Not all of which can be put down to that initial overall worry about getting older.

Thankfully the climate these days is easier and more open. And information and help are there for the asking. In the long run, knowing what may happen to you is your best protection.

SO – THE BODY IN QUESTION

There are simple tests you can have to check the levels of hormones in your body to see whether your menopause has started. But often it's self-evident and the tests just confirm what you know already.

It's thought that the difference between the women who have an easier time and those who have a tough one has to do with the rate at which oestrogen stops being produced. If oestrogen drops suddenly and dramatically, the effects can be more severe on body and mind than they are for a woman whose levels reduce more slowly. This will obviously affect women who've had their ovaries surgically removed, because then the change can be at its most abrupt.

Women who carry more fat than others often have an easier time, because fat tissues make oestrogen of their own accord. And that can ease the body's adjustment to the gradual reduction from the ovaries.

About 15 per cent of women say they have no physical side-effects from the menopause at all. It's thought they probably have very efficient adrenal glands which continue to pump out more oestrogen for longer. So for a significant spell, they have this extra 'bank' to fall back on. And when that begins to dwindle, the physical signs of menopause are often much reduced.

THE THREE STAGES

The list of symptoms may seem daunting on the face of it.

Don't let them put you off. Some are common. Some are rare. You may have only one. Or your own unique combination.

But whatever your experience, there will be a variety of remedies you can try, some of which I mention in each section, and there are others covered more fully later.

The medics break the menopause down into three distinct

phases – each with its own signs, or as they call them, symptoms.

You can bet your bottom dollar your menopause will be different in timing and length, but broadly those stages are: pre-menopausal, peri-menopausal and, you got it, post-menopausal.

The **pre-menopause** can stretch from anything between three to ten years before your actual menopause – that date of your very last period. But for most women, it's between three to four years.

The things to watch out for here are obviously irregular periods, some mood changes and hot flushes. Some people complain of headaches and dizziness, but they're not considered symptoms, though you might like to tell your doctor different. And take heart from the woman who actually found that her migraines lessened in frequency and intensity during her menopausal years.

The **peri-menopausal** phase is when you stop having periods. But that can remain a moot point for quite a long time. As we know menopause is that last and final bleeding at the very end of a woman's reproductive life. And the only way to be absolutely sure that it has happened is when you have had no periods at all for one full year.

Obviously, although you may be counting the months of what you feel is your peri-menopausal stage, it could well be that you are in the **post-menopausal** phase.

Do watch out, though. You might be having erratic periods and getting menopausal. Or you might think you are menopausal and be having what you imagine are erratic periods, and be pregnant . . .

CHAPTER 8

Penny's story

It was the haemorrhage that did it.

I've been on HRT for nine months. It's going extremely well. I never thought I'd mind that much about the wrinkles and the greying hair. But I did very much mind about the emotional and physical turmoil. Which ended up with me having the most terrible haemorrhage after six months of increasingly heavy and painful periods.

Embarrassing? The worst. The very worst moment ever. I'd got up that morning and noticed a slight bleeding. But there was no especially extra pain. Nothing unusual at all. My periods had become irregular so I just thought, oh, I'm starting another.

I went to a meeting. I'm an editor and I was getting together with the designer and the layout artist for a book I'm working on. We were at his house sitting round the table working, when I suddenly thought something wasn't right. I quickly absented myself and got myself to the loo. And there was this enormous pouring of blood. I was wearing trousers. I was soaked. They were soaked. I was absolutely terrified. It wasn't a period at all. Just blood flowing everywhere – non-stop. All over his beautiful white minimalist bathroom. The mess was terrible. I had one tampon with me. I used up all his loo paper and there still wasn't enough to absorb it.

What do you say? It was just awful. I had to go outside and explain and call my doctor. I was told to go home and lie down, and if it didn't stop to call again. And it didn't so I ended up having a scrape.

The thing is I've since heard that a lot of menopausal women go through that. Apparently it's perfectly standard. I just wish some book had mentioned it. Or I'd heard about it before. No one talks about these things.

Anyway, then I had the blood test to check my hormones and I was sufficiently low to be a candidate for HRT. I'd been saying for six months, I feel odd. Enough to feel uneasy. Strangely vulnerable emotionally. There had been physical changes too. I'd got some hairs on my chin which I'd plucked out. But now I feel a great deal better.

I have to say I remain intellectually ambivalent about HRT. There's some kind of part in me that must be the Puritan who's saying HRT's not right, and one should just take these things on the chin. But emotionally I welcome it without question.

I have a friend in her late fifties who swears by HRT. She's been on it for fifteen years. She thought she'd come off it and all her menopausal symptoms came back with a vengeance. For me, I just don't know. I guess in five years I'll go and ask somebody what the latest state of play is.

But it's a bit like *The Picture of Dorian Grey*. You think if you don't take it, you'll wake up in the morning and have aged ten years overnight.

I worry about the side-effects of HRT. The risks like cancer. But obviously not enough to stop me. You do know you're doing something artificial and there hasn't been enough time to do the research.

When *do* you stop? And *why*? And what happens then?

People's attitudes to ageing women do worry me. I'm beginning to sense a separation from younger people. And I hate that. It could just be circumstance. But it feels such a closing of a door. I loathe it. I know that something imperceptible has happened over the last year or so. I'm forty-eight and I suddenly seem to have crossed the invisible barrier. I'm not one of them any more. I'm on the other side.

Even though to yourself you're no older. Just perhaps more interesting with more good stories to tell. But not to the outside world.

I begin to see why people do things I've never had any time

for. If they're suddenly feeling like outsiders, having been inside all their lives. They're shouting, '*No. No.* I'm one of you really.'

Middle-aged people can only feel at ease with themselves if they've achieved what they'd wanted in life. More or less. Obviously there may be regrets about a few things. But if you haven't come close to your hopes and dreams and you're still trying, it's much harder.

I don't have that sense of exuberant liberation that I know that some women get at the menopause. But I think it's mainly married women who've spent their lives bringing up kids who get that. Suddenly they're free and life can change wonderfully. I'm single and childless. And I've always felt free. I've always done what I want and led the life I want so I've felt pretty free all the time.

On a practical level what's important to me now, where they weren't before, are things like wearing good clothes. And it matters that I have a good haircut. Suddenly that matters a lot.

As I look into the future I do think I have a slight anxiety about HRT. And about what would happen when I stop. Because I didn't have a good time in the six months when things were bad. I don't want to go back to that.

CHAPTER 9

The whole caboodle –

symptoms, indications, effects, side-effects,
signs and signposts to show that –yes –
this at last is it

These are some or all of the things you may experience and put down to the menopause before, during and in some cases after you've been through the three stages.

Hot flushes – or flashes; sweating and palpitations; high blood pressure; abdominal pain and 'bloating'; tiredness; nervousness; loss of concentration; dry skin; problems with teeth or gums; lack of confidence; feelings of hopelessness; moodiness; panic attacks; indecisiveness; urinary infections; loss of sex drive; loss of sexual satisfaction; aversion to being touched; headaches; insomnia; depression; irregular periods; cold feet; heavy bleeding at periods; prolapse; irritability; joint and muscle pains; dizziness; vaginal dryness; and also, less obviously and slower in its effect, a thinning of the bones may begin, osteoporosis. That's something that may not become evident until you're in your seventies.

But let's not get carried away here.

Let's pause for breath for one moment and take a look, for instance, at aching joints. That's something some women complain about at this time. But men get them too. They're usually due to physical overwork, and not related to the menopause. It's just that with a cluster of other physical sensations going on, it's hard sometimes to sort the wood from the trees. And that could be said for a number of things on that list.

As one woman said to me, 'About three years ago I got very

depressed and demoralised. I think I may have been starting the menopause. I was exhausted a lot. But I was having a terrible time at work. I hated it. And in the end simply couldn't function and decided to take early retirement.

'My life has changed. I'm so much more well adjusted. I'm happier. And now I *know* I'm right in the middle of my menopause. Unlike many women at menopause I've lost weight. But that's because I'm content with my lot and happy. So was it the beginning of the menopause then? Or was it that shitty, nasty job? I'll never know.'

FALSE START

Some women's periods stop suddenly and they think they've started the menopause, when in fact they haven't. They've got amenorrhoea. Amenorrhoea can happen from any time between puberty and the menopause and it can be the result of a number of things – not least sudden and excessive weight loss, often linked to anorexia. There may be a thyroid disorder, or a pituitary or ovarian problem.

So go to your doctor for a check-up straight away. It's unlikely to be the menopause unless you're close to the average age.

What is important, if you're having significant changes in your menstrual cycle, particularly missed periods, heavy bleeding or abdominal pain, is to see your doc. The menopause may be the culprit, but so might fibroids, cancer and other hormonal imbalances. But if you are menopausal . . .

WATCH OUT FOR

Most obviously, **irregular periods**. These usually begin in the mid- to late forties. Periods can get either more or less frequent around now. And they can become heavier or lighter than you're used to.

The ovaries are now fluctuating in their production of oestrogen and progesterone. They've been doing sterling work for many years, but the end is nigh as the two female hormones get produced more erratically.

It's now that the pituitary gland wheels into even greater action – producing more follicle-stimulating hormone to compensate. As we know, this works on the ovaries. But those sudden excess doses can force the ovary into the next cycle ahead of time.

As eventually the egg follicles respond less and less to the follicle-stimulating hormone, fewer eggs are produced. That in turn means less progesterone gets made, because progesterone is only produced once the egg has gone, leaving the empty follicle (corpus luteum) behind. It's the corpus luteum that makes the progesterone.

As we've just heard, oestrogen levels are down, but not out. Some oestrogen is still made by the ovaries and also by the adrenal glands, plus those fat cells all over the body continue to produce it.

So the oestrogen continues to do what it has always done so well – it stimulates the uterus or endometrium to expand into its sponge-like state. Without any progesterone around, it goes on doing this uninterrupted for a number of months. Which means you'll miss a period or two. And by the time the next one does get going, there'll be quite a lot of lining from the uterus to come away – hence the heavy periods. Around 30 per cent of women experience these heavy periods during their menopause.

If you're very irregular, and it's so disruptive that you want to see your GP, it's useful for you both if you go armed with a week-by-week calendar of the changing cycle so that you can both work out your pattern.

Another feature of periods at this time, whether you're in the irregular phase or not, can be a brown **discharge**, or slight **spotting** of blood leading up to, and for a few days after, a period.

Gradually over time, the gaps between periods will get

longer, weeks adding on, then months. By around your late forties or early fifties, they'll usually be over.

Some women have completely regular periods right up until their last one – when they suddenly stop.

If you're under forty and have been having signs of the menopause – if your last period was over a year ago, doctors generally agree that you are post-menopausal. If you are over forty and your last period was over a year ago, it's generally safe to stop using contraceptives. But check that out with your doc. We've all seen those widely spaced families. You get a mum, a dad and 2.5 kids trotting along quite happily for twenty-odd years till whoops – suddenly it's 3.5 kids. So watch it.

IRREGULAR BLEEDING

Irregular periods are one thing. **Irregular bleeding** is something different altogether. Irregular periods are normal. Irregular bleeding is not. It should be identified and dealt with pronto. You may have a show of blood between your periods. As your periods may already be irregular, it could be difficult for you to spot the difference. Bleeding between periods, after sex or after the menopause is over is abnormal, and needs checking out.

Irregular bleeding can be the first indication of cancer – and like most early warning signs, if acted on immediately, it can mean the difference between life and death. Many cancers are operable and an early examination can lead to 100 per cent cure.

Also
Very heavy bleeding can be exhausting and frightening. If you have to rest during your periods and your usual tampons and pads aren't adequate because of the unusually heavy flow, see the doc.

Sometimes it seems as if it never stops because the spells of bleeding are actually longer than the non-bleeding time in between. Again, it's worth getting a check-up because there are a number of possible causes.

For instance, your own oestrogen and progesterone production may very well be out of kilter and, as we've heard, could be over-stimulating the womb lining.

If you do have irregular bleeding, your doctor will want to check you for anaemia so s/he'll get the haemoglobin in your blood measured.

One cause could be **fibroids**, for which there are a number of treatments. Fibroids are extra lumps of muscle and fibrous tissue that have developed in the wall of the womb. Because they create extra surface area, they also create extra bleeding. It may be necessary to have them removed, not least to check that they are benign.

The good news is that, because of the general reduction in tissue mass around the womb at the time of menopause, many fibroids shrink quite naturally. One of the positive effects of the hormonal changes.

If none of the above is the cause of your heavy bleeding, then a course of progesterone hormones, or other drugs, can be prescribed which will stop the bleeding – but don't think that means you don't have to take contraceptive precautions, because you do.

And Another Thing
Painful periods are something even those with easy gynaecological histories get from time to time. They may increase around the menopause. But again, do get these checked out with your doctor because it could be your body sending clear messages saying, Help.

There may simply be an infection which can be easily treated with antibiotics.

Fibroids, as well as causing heavy bleeding, often increase the level of pain during the period. Again your doctor can recommend a number of courses open to you.

ENDOMETRIOSIS

The other thing that can cause unusual and treatable pain is **endometriosis**.

This gets its name from the endometrium – that spongy lining of the womb that we've already come across.

Sometimes small pieces of the womb's lining decide to go walk-about and move into other parts of the pelvic cavity, often around the ovaries, but they also lodge on the Fallopian tubes' supporting ligaments, or on the surface of the womb, bladder or bowel.

Every month, these isolated pieces of tissue do what comes naturally to them on the release of the triggering hormone – they swell and bleed. This would be all very well if this blood could in the usual way flow out of the womb and vagina along with the rest of the normal blood and tissue.

However, these pieces of tissue are deposited around the pelvis and the bleeding can't escape. It causes the kind of pain you'd get with an abscess under pressure.

The blood is partly absorbed by the body, but that which isn't can form into dark brown cysts on the ovaries. Or organs can become stuck together as scar tissue forms between them. These adhesions can cause contractions and pain in the abdomen. And even constipation, hence more pain. The pain can be at its most intense the day before a period and the first day of the period. And sometimes sex can be painful too.

Progesterone may be prescribed in the milder cases. Or a drug which stops the pituitary gland stimulating the ovary in the first place, and so stops ovulation. Which in turn means the endometrium doesn't swell and throb – in fact, it shrinks and disappears, along with the pain.

Both ovulation and menstruation will stop together. But the drug can cause side-effects, including weight gain and acne, but those go at the end of the course of treatment.

Some cases are resistant to treatment and then surgery is often the only relief.

HOT FLUSHES ...

And sweats and palpitations. Many of us have had these at some time of our adult life, usually in the first week of our period.

But for the menopausal woman they're often of a different order. They're usually at their most frequent in the two years after menopause. About 75 per cent of women get them.

They're harmless, and will eventually disappear without treatment. Their real problem is nuisance value.

They're quite unmistakable. We're not talking here about a genteel flush of the cheeks, or the becoming pink blush of a comely maiden. We're talking beetroot red from the shoulder bones up and hot, very hot, all over.

In fact, a lot of women feel hotter than they actually look. Again, some women have it worse than others. The flush, or flash, lasts for around a minute, after which there is usually sweating, followed by chill as your body temperature returns to normal.

The blood vessel network contains about sixty thousand miles, or ninety-six thousand kilometres, of capillaries. It sounds a bit like a map of the British Isles, and is probably in its way as complex and extensive. Most of the time, the capillaries on the surface of the skin are empty of blood, but during a flush they fill up and expand, giving the skin its glowing colour.

There are definite triggers to flushes, which you can try to sidestep if possible. **Stress** and **tension** are hard to avoid when you're right in the middle of them, but it certainly helps if you can lessen your load.

Alcohol, too, plus **tea** and **coffee** and some **drugs** all make the flushes worse. Unsurprisingly, they're at their most intense in **hot weather**.

The exact cause of flushes isn't known, except that they're due in some way to the combination of hormones that fluctuate in the body at menopause.

The reason they begin is that the network of tiny blood

vessels and capillaries weaving across the surface of the skin contracts. Perhaps you have a sudden emotional reaction to something. The tiniest vessels near the skin close down completely. So to begin with you go pale, as the blood is squeezed out.

Because of that, the pressure in the larger vessels leading into the capillaries goes up. The heart has to work harder to get the blood circulating back into those closed down blood vessels.

As you relax, more blood than usual is being pumped around and it flows back with force through your body's tissues, including the skin. This can be seen from the outside as you go red. At the same time you will feel warm, your blood pressure may go down, and your heart may beat faster because of the nervous system attempting to get back to normal.

The sweats that follow are a natural reaction as the body attempts to lose heat and reduce skin temperature. And the sudden drop in blood pressure can momentarily deprive the brain of sufficient oxygen to function properly, so making for brief dizzy or faint spells.

The flushes, or flashes, can be made less overwhelming. For a lot of women they're so mild that no treatment is needed. For some, they're just a mild glow. At worst, your clothes become sodden, particularly at night.

Simple things like having a cool shower instead of a bath help. Wear several layers of light clothing, even in winter, so you can discard, depending on your temperature. Nylon bras aren't good. In fact, anything nylon raises the heat level close to the body. Some hypertensive drugs increase the level of hot flushes, and your doctor may change your prescription if you're on them.

Air-conditioning isn't the answer that you might think it is. With hot flushes it's not so much rooms that are hot that need to be avoided, it's sudden changes in temperature. That seems to work as a trigger. Sudden changes in the emotions too can upset the delicate balance.

If hot flushes really are too difficult to manage, hormone replacement therapy can help (see Chapter 14). It counteracts the natural chemicals that cause instability in the blood vessels.

THOSE TWITCHY ITCHIES

Don't think you're going mad. If you suddenly feel as if you've got ants in your pants, you're not crazy. There aren't any of the actual little devils creeping round. But the sensation can be exactly the same as if there were. Just when you thought the hot flush was over, you suddenly *itch*. And it won't just be in your pants; it will be all over.

It's called **formication**, and often follows a hot flush. The word comes from the Latin *formica* which means ant. Formication is a bit like having tiny animals crawling on your skin. Irritating and uncomfortable but there's no outward sign like an eczema rash. It's not visible. It's just a physical sensation.

About fifteen to twenty per cent of menopausal women get the feeling at least once. There can also be numbness, pins and needles and tingling, all probably caused by that over-stimulation of the blood vessel network.

THE BIG BAD BLOAT

Swelling up like a balloon isn't the best way to start the day. And it gets wearying as we move around with a body that seems to expand and recede with a will of its own.

We've all had **fluid retention**, more often than not pre-menstrually, so this is something that won't be new to you, though during the menopause you may feel that it's a bit worse than usual. Again, it's those hormones changing step.

Your body can gain up to a couple of pounds a day because of fluid retention, but usually loses it at night. Shifts in the movement of body fluid occur during the day between the blood vessels and other tissues. There's much you can do to help this and we'll be looking at remedies in later chapters.

GET OUT THAT K-Y JELLY AND PARTY

Stress at any age can cause **vaginal dryness**, as can simply not being aroused by your partner. It's probably easier to treat real menopausal dryness than those first two. Menopausal dryness responds quickly to creams and lotions and potions. The first two need a good dose of the Cold Light of Day.

I can hardly bring myself to use the phrase the medics trot out for one of the most disquieting effects of the menopause – vaginal atrophy, or a dry vagina.

'Atrophy' conjures up something irreversible. And it needn't be. It sounds like the end of the world, but it is easily treatable and again is one of those things that is at its worst if ignored.

Almost everything else you go through with menopause affects you, and you alone. This affects you too. But it'll also affect your partner. It's something that needs sensitivity and tact because somehow it strikes at the very heart of our femininity, attraction and sexual pleasure.

As we know, once oestrogen levels are down, so too is the body's capacity to keep some tissues plump and moist. In fact, vaginal tissue is more dependent on oestrogen than any other part of the body. In menopause, the walls of the vagina become thin and dry. Its size can change, becoming shorter and narrower. And as muscle tone goes, it can feel looser and slacker. Vaginal secretions lessen. There's also less acid in those secretions, and as the acid protects you against yeasts and bacteria, vaginal infections can now take hold more easily.

There can be burning sensations, itching, difficulty with sex and, if there is infection, a brown or yellowish discharge.

If you've gone for a long time without sex and try it without lubrication, there may even be bleeding. The urethra and bladder can suffer. So you may have burning sensations and a more frequent need to go to the loo.

The level of symptoms may be worse for those who've had hysterectomies. A total hysterectomy, the removal of the cervix and womb, will eliminate the secretions from those areas. But if the ovaries have been removed as well, hormone levels fall too, reducing vaginal secretions even further.

One woman I spoke to had a tough time with night sweats. They were disturbing her husband, and when on top of that she noticed a change in her vagina too, she threw up her hands in horror and decided to get single beds for the two of them. The remedy doesn't have to be that drastic.

Taking longer over foreplay can help, or having sex without penetration for a while till you've found something that works for you. A simple cream can be helpful.

K-Y jelly is a good water-soluble lubricant and can be bought over the counter. And there's a new product on the market now called Replens which once put into the vagina can keep it moist for two or three days. They both couldn't be easier to use. Indeed, why not get some mileage out of a tricky transition? Turn it to your advantage. It's easy to be embarrassed at times like this, but perhaps it could actually enhance your sex life. You can each take turns applying it . . .

Pelvic floor exercises increase the flow of blood to the whole area, which could help with moisture. And natural live yoghurt put inside the vagina can soothe sore skin and ward off infections, which themselves cause dry skin.

If the soreness goes on, you can get a prescription for oestrogen creams and tablets from your doctor. Though don't apply the creams just before sex, as we don't want your partner absorbing the oestrogens as well. One person going through hormonal swings in a family is probably enough at any one time. We don't want your husband, on top of everything else, deciding it's time he started dressing up in a tutu.

THE BIG DROP

So the vaginal walls thin out. But so too do other areas of the pelvis. It's just that we're not that conscious of it. Oestrogen has been useful in maintaining pelvic tone, but some of that tone can begin to be lost. And that can affect the bladder and uterus as well as the vagina. Sometimes muscle tone goes to such an extent that they actually drop a little deeper into the pelvic region, and that's called a **prolapse**.

There's a sensation of heaviness that wasn't there before, a feeling of something moving down. Another thing you might notice, if the bladder is involved, is that coughing or laughing can lead you to involuntarily pee very slightly. It's called **stress incontinence**.

Luckily, one of the things it responds to well is exercise. Anyone who's had a baby will have come across pelvic floor exercises. The same muscles are involved here.

Surgery can also be used to repair the loosened muscles of the uterus and vagina. And that can really be of benefit if your sex life has been affected. But even then, pelvic floor exercises before and after will help you re-tone the whole area.

Pelvic Floor Exercises
If you want to try some pelvic floor exercises, lie on your back, make sure your spine is straight, and that your hips and lower back are well 'bedded into' the floor. Raise your pelvis no more than two or three inches from the ground, then lower it flat again. Repeat fifty times.

Then repeating the same tiny and controlled motion raise just the right hip fifty times, then the left fifty times. Keep the movements small.

Another exercise you can do is even more simple. Simply

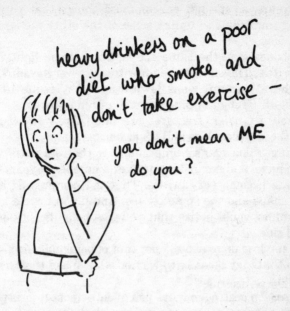

heavy drinkers on a poor diet who smoke and don't take exercise —

you don't mean ME do you?

contract and release all the muscles around your vagina. The movement is very similar to the tensing and releasing sensation you would have if you were having a pee, but were trying to release it in short bursts rather than in one long flow.

DEM BONES, DEM BONES

Sex is a good antidote to thinning of the bones, or **osteoporosis**. That's because it stimulates the adrenal glands, which at this time in your life are one of your few sources of oestrogen. So when your doctor says, 'Lead an active life and it'll help you cope with the menopause,' – s/he may be sending out subtle messages about using it, or losing it.

It is possible to keep those juices flowing. Exercise of **any** sort is great.

Bone thinning begins during the menopause and can last

many years, so it's not one of those things that you'll be noticing immediately, unlike some of the other menopausal indications.

The bones stay the same shape, but become lighter and more brittle. The signs to begin with are a very gradual loss of height. My granny went down from a statuesque 4ft 11in to about 4ft 9in by the time she died at ninety-two.

As you get older, fractures are more likely to occur, so watch those wrists, legs and lower backs.

Getting a dowager's hump is one of the real fears many women have, and it can develop over a number of years if the vertebrae become very brittle. They get compressed into a wedge shape and the spine curves. And if you have a stroke or an injury you'll notice that you lose bone density on the injured side.

You can lose up to about 1 per cent of bone mass each year, though that may be more in women who've had their ovaries removed.

The reason oestrogen helps you avoid osteoporosis is that it helps to prevent calcium from being lost from your bones. Calcium both builds and maintains your skeleton, and without oestrogen to keep it in the body, you excrete it in your urine.

Heavy drinkers lose more bone mass than others. So do people on a poor diet and those who don't take exercise.

Luckily, these are all things we can do something about.

CHAPTER 10

Phew! What a catalogue of varying calamities!

I can't stress enough that not all women will have all these indications at all times of the menopause.

Something that seems minor to one, will be more problematic to another. Some will remain strangers to them all.

I've time and again come across medics who are very rigid in their definition of what exactly they consider true symptoms of oestrogen deficiency, or the menopause.

To the rest of us with our aches and twinges and sudden unexplainable lurgies, everything that smacks of pain and inconvenience at that 'certain time of life' can oh, so easily get lumped under the same umbrella.

Don't forget men age too. And they age because that is what the body does naturally. As yours does, with or without the menopause. As it has been doing before, and as it will after. Not everything is caused by that sudden, or gradual, loss of the female hormones.

Strictly speaking, some medics would take me to task for including some of the things I have in the above list. A lot of them would have been happy if I had included only the following: loss of periods, hot flushes and night sweats.

That's your lot. These they consider true oestrogen-deficiency symptoms.

To quote one, and I'm reluctant to because I hate the jargon, but to repeat what he says, the rest are 'psycho-socio-cultural symptoms'. I'm sure he knows where he can park that lot.

On the other hand, another doc I talked to relentlessly

47

listed twenty-one different symptoms that she claimed were linked directly to the menopause. By their own lights they're both probably right. It's just a question of naming, categorising and prioritising. Some things must be dealt with immediately. Others will pass with patience.

Whatever they want to call it, what is important is that you get treated for anything that you think needs treating. And that you get help and advice on things you can do for yourself.

Another thing is not to lose perspective about what's really going on. If you've just read the previous pages in one sitting, that might be a little difficult. But bear with me.

Physical symptoms are real and at times uncomfortable. Their effect on a woman's life should never be denied.

But something else is just as important. And that something is attitude. A lot of the way we experience our menopause depends so much on how we feel about it. How we feel about ourselves. How we feel about our place in the world. What's going on with our life at the moment. Work. Family. Love. Loss. Change.

So, having looked at the body – next, it's the mind.

CHAPTER 11

Brave new world

'I'm sure as hell not having a bunch of men look at a woman who no longer has eggs and saying, "You're not viable, babe!" '

Sock it to 'em, Lauren. The glorious Lauren Hutton, American model and actress, has always had a big mouth. And she's not backward about coming forward with what's on her mind. She's a big brave lady who's not afraid to tell the truth. Given her profession, you'd think the safest thing for her would be to stay quiet and keep taking the money for as long as they pay her. But she's on a crusade. She's confronting America's attitude to women and ageing head-on.

She's fifty. She's drop-dead gorgeous. And she's just signed an enormous contract with Revlon. She was famous twenty years ago for being the highest-paid model then. Well, at age fifty she's just personally negotiated a second deal with Revlon for more money than she made in the first.

I know she has the looks of one in a million. But she means what she says. She's had a clause written into all her photographic contracts headed 'no-retouch'. It forbids the use of the airbrush on any of her pics. There's nothing wrong with plastic surgery. But she's decided to take a stand and tell it like it is. Lines, wrinkles, bags, sags and all. 'I don't want to look like an egg,' she says. 'I *used* to, but I don't want to any more.'

And women like it. She says that women in their middle years come up to her and thank her for just being there. For affirming that women 'of a certain age' not only exist, but are 'viable'.

With or without eggs.

And that hits the nail on the head. Do we really only get our social affirmation from being a walking egg-bank? What is it about being fertile that makes a woman more 'viable'? Because the brutal truth of the matter is that in the Western world, that's just the way it is.

Youth has the drive and energy. Youth sells product. Youth dominates our world view. Show me an advert for an unassuming, rather ordinary bar of chocolate and I'll show you a juicy, nubile girl licking something phallic. And enjoying it. Sex-equals-youth-equals-pleasure. Sex-equals-social visibility-equals-power. By the time she gets to menopause, a woman is dealing with attitudes inscribed on the other side of that coin.

We may think we've got a sensible, no-nonsense approach to ageing, but scratch the surface, and deep down many of us are bound with fears. And it's not surprising. The climate isn't so great out there once you get past your sell-by date.

Agreed, you only have to look around you to see thriving, busy, middle-aged women leading creative and full lives. So you may argue that the dragon has been laid to rest. But those fears, irrational as they're increasingly being proven to be, are still lurking and pulsing just beneath the surface.

One GP I spoke to told me of her own personal experience. She's particularly sensitive about treating menopausal women and values that part of her practice – maybe because she's a woman. Maybe because she's a good doctor. Maybe because she had an early menopause at forty.

Whatever the reason, she cares. Her own menopause shocked her. It came early. And was so unexpected. Plus she had qualified as a doctor unusually late.

'I felt, just a minute,' she said, 'I've only just got going. And suddenly it's all over. I haven't even started doing some of the things I want to do.' She's a particularly dynamic woman who had a vision about her work and her many ambitions.

'Somehow – the two things became one. I was no longer "fertile" and it didn't seem to be only a physical infertility. I felt it touched every part of my life. It wasn't only the ability to recreate with my body. It meant my creative intellectual life was also over. Somehow losing the one meant I'd lost the drive and potency in the other too.'

So here we have a doctor, a woman who more clearly than most of us knows there's no link between physical infertility and the mind, confusing the two. For one brief muddled moment in her life, mind and body were intimately and inextricably linked. Being 'infertile' weakened her. Somehow she felt sidelined from the more 'fruitful' world she had been part of up till then.

Needless to say, it passed. And she has gone on to write the books she planned, carve out the career she worked so long and hard for, and contribute in a way she'd always wanted to. But it's an indication of how very easy it is to buy into social attitudes that in no way reflect our own personal experience.

Twenty-seven per cent of husbands have no idea what their wives are going through at the menopause. And if twenty-seven per cent don't know *anything*, then there must be many, many more who have only the sketchiest idea. It's not something that needs to be proclaimed to the four corners of the world. But if even partners are in the dark, doesn't that smack of shame and embarrassment?

There's nothing quite so stark as the difference between the image of a healthy, contributing, reproductive member of the species and that of a dried-up old crone. That may sound harsh, but peel away the layers of sophisticated civilisation and what you get is a primitive gut response. Lack of fertility means uselessness. In the eyes of the tribe, uselessness means death. Intellectually we may pooh-pooh such nonsense. But our instincts tell us different.

And that's why women like Lauren Hutton are so important. And there are many like her. Maybe not so public. Many leading quiet, private existences. But strong women nevertheless who are saying, 'Take me as you find me. I'm staying right here – middle age and all. I will not crawl away and die.'

51

There's a complex interchange between the way a woman sees herself, and the way society sees her. Some societies reward women when they reach the menopause. Others punish. Western society carries some of the most negative attitudes of all.

In some countries women experiencing menopause have had measurably less pain and discomfort *with the same symptoms* than women elsewhere.

In some countries the menopause is a blessing. Positive attitudes to it seem to have reduced physical problems.

In many African tribes, it's only after women have finished their years of being lowly bearers of children and drawers of water that they are allowed to take a place of full social and political equality in the village hierarchy. Finally they can join their male contemporaries and take part fully with the voting and decision making.

These women positively welcome the menopause.

The same goes for a number of Arab countries. Again it is women in their fertile years who don't seem to be fully realised social beings. Some Muslim women will not go into a room with a man in it if they are menstruating. Menstrual blood is considered defiling. I know a British girl born and brought up here in the Church of England who married a Kuwaiti and whenever she returns to this country she will not speak to, or be in the same room as, her father for one week out of every four.

However, as soon as the evidence of full-blooded sexuality has gone, so too do the social restrictions.

The women of the Rajput in India also experience fewer menopausal symptoms and actively look forward to menopause, because that's when they come out of purdah. Again their social standing rises.

The irony of these examples, of course, is that these women are still being tyrannised for their sexuality; it's simply in reverse. However, they are striking indications of the way in which all our lives are shaped by the societies we are born into. Current sexual 'status' is always the dominant measure.

No wonder the women in those countries felt better at menopause, and had fewer problems. They were probably too busy finally joining the mainstream of the human race.

The social stigma in the West can lead to very real anxieties. In their book, *Menopause: a Time for Positive Change*, Fairlie, Nelson and Popplestone recount a telling tale about a woman terrified of the approaching 'change'.

She had an inkling that her menopause might be starting as she was beginning to have slightly irregular periods. But more important to her than anything else was that her hair was beginning to fall out. She was convinced it was because of the menopause. Was she right? And was she going to go bald? She was sure she had heard it was a symptom.

This was notwithstanding the fact that a number of women in her family had already lost a lot of hair, and were going bald themselves after being diagnosed as having the nervous disorder, alopecia.

Alopecia leads to partial or complete baldness and has nothing to do with the menopause whatsoever.

But she was still sure it did. Once she was told she was wrong, that her hair loss was simple straightforward baldness, unrelated in any way to the menopause, she felt much, much better. The baldness didn't really seem to matter to her at all. What did matter was being somehow publicly identified, because of her baldness, as menopausal.

Do we in the UK suffer more actual physical pain and psychological upheaval because we're going through the same thing as those women in other societies – but in reverse? For us, there's no carrot at the end of the road. Just an uncomfortable, unspoken but all-pervading feeling that the best is over. Only the worst is yet to come.

CHAPTER 12

Running into the buffers?
Or fast-tracking to a new life?

We absorb the attitudes around us. Subtly and not so subtly, we learn to take our place in the scheme of things. We can take those attitudes on board – which means colluding and agreeing with them – or we can confront them, which will inevitably work towards change.

Even as we deal with society's ties that bind, we have to cope with the tiny dramas of our own lives, the personal and the intimate.

If the attitudes of society can affect us so much, then how much more will our own life experiences also have a bearing?

If a woman planned a life for herself that included satisfying work, marriage, three happy, healthy children and a lifelong partnership with a devoted husband – and fate *delivered* exactly that, she's likely to approach the menopause with a degree of equanimity.

But for the woman who hoped for more or less the same, and got instead a fractured career, two broken marriages, two abortions and a miscarriage, plus the loss of the most important love affair of her life at around the age of forty-one and a half – menopause will probably be an altogether more bitter pill.

Having just covered the physical aspects of the menopause, I am mindful of how concrete and overwhelming they can be. And that's something never to lose sight of.

And yet, so very important too are our own attitudes and expectations. The way we choose to sail across the sometimes choppy waters of this transition time can make all the difference between staying afloat, or going under.

In 1991 a research project called the Massachusetts Womens' Health Study found that from among three thousand women, the majority of those who said they felt emotionally negative about their periods ending had more painful physical symptoms than those with a more positive attitude.

Many approach this time in their lives positively. For some it's a true liberation, and not just for those who never wanted children at all. For mothers, it can be a timely end to a fruitful but long chapter of caring and nurturing. Now is the time to begin anew. A time perhaps to focus on their own needs. A time to find more time for themselves.

It can be a blessed release to be free of the rigmarole of contraception. It may coincide with children growing up and leaving home. It may come as a welcome time of general reassessment. A pause. A taking stock. Partnerships can change. Sex can change too, once the emphasis is no longer on childbearing, or rearing. Menopause could be a springboard to the best years of your life.

Positive thinking has real payoffs. According to a Healthy Women's Study at the University of Pittsburgh in 1991, women who thought that learning the facts about menopause and maintaining an upbeat attitude would help them, had an easier time of it. They had lower levels of depression and fewer symptoms overall than women with pessimistic outlooks.

Easier said than done, but it's something to mull over.

I came across an example of positive thinking just the other day, while I was working on this book. I phoned a specialist medical research library to double check the scope of their medical journals. I had expected a thirty-second conversation but it didn't quite go like that.

Nice Lady Who Picked Up the Phone: 'Hello. British Library Science Reference Section.'

Me: 'Hello. I'm doing some research and I just wanted to check that you've got some medical journals that I want to read. To see if they're actually on your premises now.'

Nice Lady: 'Well, it depends what you're researching. *If* for instance it's research into the menopause you're doing, we've most things here. Or we can get them.'

Me: (In a state of some surprise – forgetting for the moment any interest in technical data) 'Er. Um. Well, yes, actually, it's strange you should say that. As it happens, I am doing research into the menopause.'

(Pause)

(Silence)

Me: (Mindful this could be a minefield and mindful I could be being extremely rude) 'You're not, er, um, going through it yourself, are you?'

Nice Lady: 'Yes, I am.'

Me: 'Er. Um. How's it going for you?'

From which followed ten minutes of conversation about her own personal experiences, with me saying very little. Talking about it seemed positively beneficial. I got a real sense that this was an important part of her process, and of her making sense of what she was going through. It had value. It warranted recognition. As did the way she was managing it.

And it was clear she was having quite a tough time of it. But somehow she was keeping it in proportion:

'It's a matter of remembering you're getting older. Things are just not the same. We all think we'll last forever. That we're not going to slow down.

'I've had hot flushes. I had them every ten minutes day and night. They never seemed to stop. I'd wake up gasping. That's if I got to sleep. I'd have to throw off the bedclothes. The worst thing is I was so tired. Not because of the hot flushes themselves. But because I couldn't sleep.

'The thing is you know it's not going to go on forever. You've just got to grin and bear it. It does pass.

'And I've never been one for all that alternative medicine stuff. But I've been taking vitamin B6 and that helps. And Evening Primrose Oil, and that helps too. I don't know if it's a coincidence but I haven't had a night sweat in the three months since I started. I take them because I know they can't hurt me. I wouldn't take just anything. The doctor gave me some pills. I don't know what they were. But they didn't do anything.

'The thing is you have to get your mind geared to say to yourself you *are* going to change. Give in. Gracefully. And do the best you can. You can't stop the clock.

'There are so many different things you have to cope with. This gets thrown at you in a time in your life when you think you're all settled. But then everything comes at once. And it usually comes when you don't need it.

'When you talk to other women about it, you always hear something worse. It's awful. But it makes you feel better.

'Every day is different. There are good days and bad days. When I get up I just hope it's going to be a good day.'

A sixth sense told me that, strangely enough, for all her candour it would be the height of impertinence for me to ask her what her name was. Now that *was* personal. We parted cordially, with me sobered and impressed.

There was a great determination running through her conversation. She raised a number of issues that I'll be looking at in later chapters – self-help, alternative medicines, hormone replacement therapy.

But what I want to focus on here was her attitude. It's clear she hadn't had an easy time of it, and indeed there were still good days and bad days. But though at times she seemed to be entirely subject to her body's whims and caprices, there was a willingness to ride it. It would pass.

No one has the right to make a judgement about how others choose to negotiate difficult times. We each have to live our lives in our own way. But the facts do seem to say that attitude of mind can turn a bad experience around. It may not go away but it no longer completely overwhelms.

However, it is hard to reshape attitudes. A very good woman counsellor confided that, even though she is trained to be psychologically acute and informed, she was in denial about the menopause. It's not surprising the rest of us find it hard to shift the occasional 'resistance' or 'block'. We're all busy dealing with what is immediate in our lives. Our time is full enough without spending it on something that's part of a rather improbable, faintly unpleasant, nebulous future.

I'm sure a lot of this denial comes from fear. Menopause hasn't had a good press.

One woman told me how she remembers her mother as perfectly balanced and happy through her childhood, but as soon as she hit those 'uncertain years' she had suffered a severe depression. In those days, and we're talking thirty-five years ago when the medical world was both woefully ignorant, and woefully unsympathetic, she was diagnosed as 'menopausal' and given electric shock therapy. And after THAT she was put on a daily dose of tranquillisers. Doctors really did not know then how addictive Mother's Little Helpers could be. At the age of 75, she is still on them. I asked what her life is like now.

'Well,' said the woman, 'she sleeps a lot. Morning. Noon. And night.'

Given a history like that, is it surprising that her daughter approaches her middle years, just a touch nervous?

Luckily these days so much more is known about the menopause. There is so much more than can be done to help. And one enormous stride is in the development and refinement of hormone replacement therapy.

CHAPTER 13

Ingrid's story

You do strange things. That's one of the first signs, apart from the obvious physical ones.

And I was inordinately tired. And I'm only forty-eight. Occasionally before, if I had bad PMS I'd take a quick nap in the afternoon. But now it was every afternoon, around three or four. I'd just have to lie down for twenty minutes. We were using the flat as an office so I could do it.

In fact, everything in life became like one long PMS symptom. The confusion, the irritability. The tearfulness. Terrific mood swings. It's a swine. I'm being dragged through it kicking and screaming.

Along with it came a subtle shift in personality. I felt more negative. My husband would come in with new business dreams and schemes and I used to be able to be positive. Now it just all seemed like a load of shit.

It was a vague depression on a permanent basis. Real pessimism. No matter what was offered me, I just felt an underlying discontent. Men don't understand. Even women don't understand. They think you're a negative old carping woman who's no fun to be around.

After about the first two or three months I had the first realisation that this was what ageing is. Till then I'd moved like a young person. Thought like a young person, and had a feeling of invincibility. Suddenly I felt vulnerable. I was no longer eternally youthful, beautiful, powerful, able. There was a part of me that had felt free from any constrictions at all. Then came this gut realisation I was part of the whole pattern of things and could and would be moved about like a piece on a chessboard. Without my say-so.

59

I was suddenly an older, wiser, more settled and *dumpy* middle-aged lady.

And maternal. I felt I was like my mother. And that's bad. Because I was *never, ever* going to be like my mother.

I sat differently. I moved differently. I used to sit with my legs thrown over the side of a chair, swinging my feet. Or up on the table. Suddenly I was sitting with my knees together, like a lady.

And my sex drive was gone. I used to be rampant. And it's faded. That led to dumb resignation. I thought, oh God, no. Not this too. Along with the grey hair and drying skin, crabbiness. It was as though I'd run into a brick wall that said *old age*. It's been my first serious confrontation.

I'm forty-seven now, but I'd say it's been subtly building since my early forties. My memory's been getting more erratic for the last eight years or so. My sister has had the same symptoms. And she's so much more accepting. I admire women like that. English women just seem to get on with it. I don't know how they do it. Not me. And I do think there are a whole horde of us crabby critters out there.

The confidence in your femininity goes. Those of us who've used our wiles to their fullest knew they were powerful. And suddenly that weapon is no longer available. I don't mean in terms of battle – but it's just a useful tool to get through life. And it's gone. If your car broke down you'd smile sweetly at the man at the garage. Now if you go up to the same guy, you imagine he's saying, 'Christ, what does this old bat want?'

There's a mental confusion. A lowered level of concentration. And shocking memory loss. I've left passports in airports. Lost keys. Lost the car. Thought I was going senile and developing Alzheimer's.

And along with that, a lowered interest in the world at large. I used to read a number of newspapers regularly, and periodicals and things. Now I don't have the inclination.

And all of this was *before* I had my first hot flushes and night sweats. Which are the really classic symptoms.

I had an urge to commit suicide. It kind of drifted in and out like a vague fog. My ability to cope with stress shrank dramatically. And when I did have stressful situations I reacted more negatively. I couldn't cope.

This whole lot lasted over a two-year period. But it started so subtly. I wasn't aware. It gradually gained momentum in the last six months. Then it got real bad.

I felt like Frankenstein's monster. As if there were two screws either side of my forehead – and someone somewhere was tightening them all the time. The same for my whole spine, which felt as if a corkscrew was twisting it into a permanent spiral. I could easily have murdered.

By the end of the six months I was a basket case and Philip insisted I go to the doctor who immediately put me on HRT. Within days the tearfulness and extreme irritability had gone.

I felt more me. As if I was coming back from a long way away. I was more in control. I could remember where I'd put my bag. I didn't feel like a cork bobbing hopelessly in the sea. The demon was no longer in charge.

And at the same time I just feel a genuine sense of grief and frustration at the unfairness of it all. Now as soon as I get jumpy again, Philip immediately asks me if I've taken my pill. He's terrified that gorgon will return.

I don't know if it's a magic cure-all. I don't care. It worked and it continues to work.

I've been on it four months and I'll stay on HRT till I can find a suitable substitute. It seems to help so many psychological things. And then things like my hair. And my skin. My husband had to go and identify the body of a friend of ours who died. He always had springy, curly hair. Philip said it was the one thing that looked different about him. It had gone flat and lank. That's how mine went too.

And my sex drive is back. Not 100 per cent but it's better. And also I'm thrilled to be still having regular periods. I like that. I don't mind bleeding every month. It's a cycle that feels natural and good. I like being part of it.

I feel a different woman. I'm still desperately trying to

hang on to the old one. I'm determined to for as long as I can. But we all need more information. You know they say age is all in the mind. Well, let me tell you I have sore knees, an aching hip, pain in my back and I'm often stiff all over. Life slows down. If I do any exercise these days I have to start very slowly. I never had to do that before.

And let me also tell you there are women who go through worse. Philip has been behind me 100 per cent. He cares. Other women have to go through all this. Then their husband runs off with the secretary. Or their mother becomes senile. Or their daughter gets divorced. Or their husband has a mad business scheme combined with his own mid-life crisis and they lose all their money. I wail and mourn for the women of the world. The worst things happen just when you can't cope.

I feel now that I'm at a crossroads. I'm looking round at alternatives to taking HRT long-term. I'm grateful and thankful that more research is being done. They will find better ways to relieve the symptoms. And I know I've got to make the best of it.

CHAPTER 14

The debate – HRT: to go for it, or run a mile?

'It was bliss. Within weeks I was almost back to normal. No more weeping. No wailing. And more energy. Much more energy.'
Sarah, forty-five.

'I wouldn't touch it with a barge-pole. I don't care how long I have to put up with these hot flushes. It's just not natural.'
May, forty-seven.

There you have it. Those two women couldn't be further apart. One swears by hormone replacement therapy. The other thinks it's a kind of madness.

To take HRT, or not to take HRT? It can be one of the toughest decisions.

Doctors themselves are divided. So where does that leave us as consumers? We know the medics disagree over the precise symptoms of the menopause. The menopause is recognised as that time in a woman's life when there is a gradual reduction of oestrogen. That in its turn may cause hot flushes, vaginal dryness and osteoporosis, or a weakening of the bones.

But some doctors would like to increase that list to include headaches, dizziness, aching joints, mood swings and much more. The purists stick to the first three.

As one doctor said to me, 'You really do have to make a distinction between deciding that you are treating the menopause, pure and simple, and not all the related side-effects of simply growing old.

'Yes, women have oestrogen deficiency. And yes, women grow old. But these can be parallel states. They're not always directly linked. The best you can do is gen up on as much information as you can, so that whatever choice you do make, at least you know the pros and cons.'

ETERNAL YOUTH V. MONKEY GLAND ADDICTION

First, let's junk those myths. The hormones used in HRT are not made from monkey glands. But they are 'natural'. The oestrogen used in most HRT products originates from the urine of pregnant mares. The most commonly prescribed is called premarin. 'Pre' for pregnant, 'mar' for mare, and 'in' for urine.

The compounds used mimic the female hormones in the human body. As the ovaries produce less, HRT steps in and

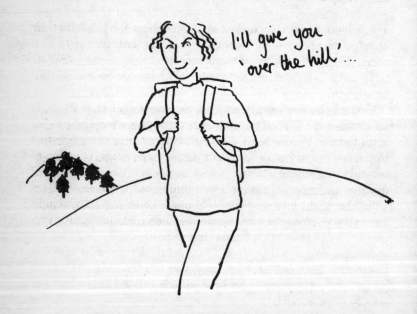

I'll give you
'over the hill'...

starts doing the work for them. And that keeps the reproductive system ticking over at a time when it would otherwise go into natural decline.

HRT does not promise eternal youth. It is not a ticket for the carpet ride to the never-never land of Shangri-La where people never age.

What it does seem to do for some is even out the mood swings brought on by fluctuating hormonal supplies. In the long term it seems to protect those prone to either osteoporosis or coronary heart disease. In the short term it eases the hot flushes, maintains skin tone, and vaginal dryness disappears. Oestrogen encourages the body to retain fluid; this can puff out the skin and stretch it, and so seem to reduce wrinkles.

But it doesn't make you twenty-one again. And it doesn't stop ageing.

It may *feel* as if the clock has been thrown into reverse. But that's often because a woman has been having difficult physical symptoms to contend with, and the relief when they are gone is so immense that she's temporarily lost sight of where normal comes on the gauge.

One doctor I spoke to said it is absolutely not proven that it helps with depression and anxiety, which are some of the claims:

'There is no evidence. But once you've got the hot flushes out of the way, and vaginal dryness, a woman's morale is so much better. You've got rid of the two key things. A woman may have to get up a number of times each night to change not only her nightie, but her sheets too. Because they're literally soaking. Of course she's depressed. And tired. Get rid of the night sweats and she'll get a proper night's sleep. Naturally you're going to see more of a sparkle in her eyes.'

HOW TO TAKE IT

There are a number of ways to take HRT, but the two most popular are by **pill**, or by transdermal application – known as **'the patch'** to you and me.

Implants of HRT are used most often by women who have had their ovaries and womb removed. A hormone pellet is inserted into the fatty tissue of the wall of the stomach under local anaesthetic and should usually last around six months. Two problems are that sometimes they don't last that long. And if there are side-effects it's almost impossible to find them again and get them out.

Pessaries are also used mainly for women who've had surgery. Placed in the sensitive skin of the vagina, they're absorbed quickly and can be helpful with vaginal problems. The vagina absorbs so well that oestrogen applied there could overstimulate the womb for those women who, because they still have their wombs and ovaries, are having a natural menopause.

THE PATCH OR THE PILL?

The principle for each remains the same, but you tend to get more oestrogen into the body with the *pill*. It's taken once a day. The digestive system absorbs it, the blood-stream transports it round the body, then it goes to the liver to be eliminated. The oestrogen works in tandem with the body's natural chemicals and as an extra bonus actually helps produce some substances that have positive side-effects.

Some women like taking the pill, but it shouldn't be used by everyone. The hormones in it are natural, and one of the features of a natural hormone is that it doesn't dissolve easily in water. So some women may be taking the pill every day, but they can't digest it.

Other women with liver disease, gall-bladder disease or

blood-clotting disorders should steer clear of HRT. But that's something that'll be clearly identified by your doctor.

The HRT pill is popular because the breakthrough bleeding of the period is controlled. And it is cheap.

'The patch' is the latest technique and is the favourite with a lot of women. Each patch contains the necessary dose of hormone, and it's simply applied to the skin, usually of the hip, thigh or abdomen. Oestrogen is released directly into the bloodstream in a steady, constant dose.

One woman told me the only thing she didn't like about it was that it collected bits of fluff and looked dirty. If you had a new lover and didn't want them to know you were on HRT, you had to take it off. And then it left a red welt on your skin. But in terms of delivering oestrogen, it worked.

Some women find that they need a higher dose of oestrogen when using the patch than they did when taking the pill. But a study carried out in Milan in 1989 showed that women who use the patch quickly get greater control over their hot flushes than those who are taking oestrogen orally.

The patch is a popular method because smaller doses are necessary, and it doesn't affect blood pressure. It's also useful if there are digestive problems. The downside is that the patch sometimes falls off, reducing effectiveness; bleeding patterns aren't so predictable, and it is expensive.

BUT IT TAKES TWO TO TANGO, SO WHAT ABOUT PROGESTERONE?

So far all we've heard about is oestrogen. But as we know, there are two stars to this show. The oestrogen works on building muscle tissue in the first half of the menstrual cycle. The progesterone then steps in and triggers the process that clears the lining of the womb at the end.

Most women who take the oestrogen part of HRT, unless

they've had a hysterectomy, also need to take progesterone. Without progesterone, the uterus is eventually bombarded with too much oestrogen. That means it never gets the benefit of the flushing and cleansing process of the second female hormone, progesterone.

If HRT has a bad reputation, it may be because when it was prescribed back in the early days, only oestrogen was used. That meant a lot of women experienced excessive growth of the womb's lining. That's called hyperplasia, and is a precancerous condition. There was a time when women on HRT seemed to suffer a greater risk of womb cancer. A lot of fear about HRT stems from then.

It's possible these days to target the combination therapy more precisely to each woman's needs, though almost all doctors are agreed that however much of either drug they prescribe – less is best.

The amount you're prescribed will generally be in line with the amounts your body generated naturally in your premenopausal days. That's why some doctors do tests on you earlier than you might think necessary, just so they can have a record of what's needed later. If there is no record, then you may both need to experiment till you find the dose that feels comfortable.

CYCLES

HRT can be taken in such a way that you'll apparently go on having your normal menstrual cycle. You won't have a real period where an unfertilised egg is lost – it's artificially created withdrawal bleeding, clearing out the lining of the womb, and probably won't be as heavy as your periods used to be. If you are taking the **pill**, with some makes you stop taking them entirely for a week during the withdrawal bleeding.

The **patch** is effective for about three days, so you change it about twice-weekly. Again, as with the pill you will get the regular bleeding.

IS IT GOING TO DO ME ANY HARM?

'I've had the box of pills in the medicine cabinet for three months and just can't bring myself to begin. The thing is I have such a strong reaction to begin with, I have to clear the decks socially, and then set a whole weekend aside doing nothing because it's so strong.'
Worried consumer.

Some people have a bad reaction to HRT and find, ironically, that while taking it they get all the PMS symptoms, but without the relief. For them it just doesn't work.

A lot of their fears and anxiety stem from a general mistrust that it's going against nature. It's not natural. The body should be left to its own devices and it'll all sort out in the end.

And as we've heard, HRT was for some time associated with higher risks of cancer. This worries many, not least as one GP said, because, 'As with all things, risks make headlines and benefits do not.'

Another GP ran his own mini-survey for me on the patients in his practice and of the menopausal women he was seeing, 53 per cent in their mid-forties were on HRT, or had at some time tried it. That tallies with general estimates of the women who chose to try it out during menopause.

If it works for you, it can bring immense relief very quickly. 'Sometimes they think I'm going to take them off it,' he went on, 'and they get really alarmed and say, "Please don't make me stop." They quite literally bounce in and say, "I'm a new woman." '

'It's better than a G and T,' says another happy user. 'Last week my husband backed my car into the gatepost and I just laughed. It would have been a different scenario six months ago.'

Another told me, 'I felt like I was at the bottom of a deep pit. It was complicated by the fact that looking back I reckon my menopause started at thirty-eight. But because I was so young no one else reckoned it was. Till finally I had one of those hormone level tests and my oestrogen was way, way down. And must have been for years. I thought I was an insomniac for four years. As soon as I started taking HRT I could sleep.

'Normally you can juggle twenty things at once. Suddenly it's all too much. One little hormonal imbalance and you'll shoot your partner, or jump out of the window. I think one day they're going to discover that oestrogen is the secret of life.'

Sylvie was one of those from the 'stick with Mother Nature' group. She had always gone down the complementary medicine path. She swore she'd never touch HRT. But when the menopause arrived she was unlucky. It hit hard. She was having to do a lot of travelling to support her husband's business ventures world-wide. The disruption and dislocation were unsettling, and she found she was increasingly exhausted.

And more important than that, she was unable to draw on the extra reserves she'd always been able to in previous stressful times. Some people would say it was just that she wasn't getting any younger. Others that the romance of international jet lag had worn off and her heart just wasn't in it, as it had been when they were both hungry and setting up the business. Whatever it was, 'It' was all getting too much.

Then one day she found she was in Paris, in the middle of winter, with just T-shirts, trousers and about thirty-five pairs of shoes in her suitcase – all her winter clothes were in storage somewhere on the last continent she'd transited. Some madwoman had packed her bags all wrong, and she had to suppose that must have been her. She had a complete brainstorm. She sat down and started crying and didn't stop for about three months. Eventually her partner got her to go to the doctor who immediately prescribed HRT.

Within days she began to feel, and look, like her old self. She doesn't like being on HRT. But neither did she like what went before.

As I said, it's not an easy choice for some. But many women

swear by it and wouldn't be without.

HOW LONG, OH LORD, HOW LONG?

'I've found women keep taking it till they've "medicalised" themselves enough,' says one GP. 'They come off it themselves, but I've noticed that if they have the same symptoms as when they went on HRT, they're back on it like a shot.

'It's a bridge – not a postponement. When you come off HRT, you return to a body which is at exactly the same stage it would have been if you'd never taken HRT. If you were due to have hot flushes for two years and you take HRT for eighteen months, they'll still be there when you come off. If you decide to keep going for three years, they'll be gone by the time you stop.

'You have to experiment for a bit. And it's different for every woman.'

Some doctors say you've got to take it till the day you fall off your perch. Being brutally frank, one doctor told me, 'If you're a candidate for osteoporosis, taking HRT for ten years can postpone your fracture from when you're seventy to when you're eighty years old.' Doctors who are prescribing HRT to prevent osteoporosis, advise taking it for a minimum of ten to fifteen years.

Some doctors recommend only three to five years, with a reduction in the dosage towards the end. They're concerned mainly with treating immediate physical effects such as osteoporosis and coronary heart disease, more of which later.

The point is it's a new therapy. One doctor who prescribes both responsibly and with constant monitoring, used the words 'chronic' therapy when talking about it to me.

When I said, 'Chronic?' he replied, 'Yes. You're taking a lot of drugs, for a long time. Whatever else you call it, and however harmless, that's a chronic treatment. You can give patients a chronic therapy of drugs for the short term and their bodies can throw off the toxic effects once they come off them. The body can cope with that.

'But it hasn't been possible to do really long-term studies on HRT, because the drugs themselves just haven't been in general use that long. We don't know what the cumulative effects are over a long period. The experiment's still in progress. The jury's still out.'

And most patients as well as doctors will tell you that though HRT gets rid of tiresome menopausal symptoms, it can be at a price.

THE BAD NEWS

You may have side-effects when taking HRT, some of which are temporary and will ease of their own accord within months of starting treatment. Some don't go, but can be helped with diet and exercise. All of them fade as soon as you stop.

They can include cramps, tender breasts, bloating, queasiness, weight gain and headaches.

Cramps have to be put up with in much the same way as when you were having your natural periods. You're taking technically the same hormones, and they're doing the same thing as your own hormones will have done. Relaxing exercises and herbal teas can help.

One of the most common effects of HRT is **bloating**. Around 50 per cent of women get it. Oestrogen encourages the body to absorb and retain more salt than is necessary. Salt in its turn attracts and retains water, so the body tissues swell. Some doctors prescribe diuretics. But just reducing your salt intake and cutting down on caffeine helps.

If you were always prone to **headaches** and **migraines**, these may continue and increase. Again, it's due to fluid retention. Even the brain can swell up. Some women have to decide which is worse, the menopausal symptoms or the migraines. But on the other hand, some women find their migraines get better on HRT.

Around 25 per cent of women gain **weight**, especially at the beginning of their HRT treatment. This can also be put down to fluid retention, and it usually disappears once the body has adjusted to the new HRT balancing act. Some women put on weight because they've got to a time in their life when they exercise less and their metabolism has slowed down. It's easy to confuse the two.

SPOT CHECKS AND REGULAR SERVICES

Get monitored regularly, thoroughly and often
As long as you're taking the juice, you should be regularly checked out.

First of all, to fine-tune your dosage. To begin with, you've got to work out what's exactly right for your body. Your metabolism, your lifestyle and your physical condition are all unique to you. There may be a bit of a trial and error as you and your doc experiment for a while finding the right dose, which is high enough to relieve your symptoms, but low enough to stay safe over the long term.

It can take three or four months. During that time if your breasts get very tender, or you notice a vaginal discharge and you feel more bloated than usual, your dosage is probably too high.

If the dose is too low, then you'll just go on feeling the same menopausal symptoms that you're trying to get rid of.

THE RISKS

The other reason you need to be monitored is that HRT does carry risks. Menopausal women are grateful when oestrogen supplements relieve vaginal dryness and night sweats, and protect them against osteoporosis.

But oestrogen doesn't just work on those isolated areas. Its effects are more widespread. It travels to the liver, the heart, the uterus, the ovaries and the breasts, and sometimes it can cause damage. So do have pelvic and breast check-ups, including the usual routine mammograms and pap smears at the appropriate time.

If you're over fifty, you should be having those every three years *anyway*, whether you're on HRT or not.

And if **endometrial or womb cancer** runs in your family, your doctor may decide to do an endometrial biopsy, particularly if you have irregular vaginal bleeding.

Oestrogen has been labelled the bad guy in the rise in levels of endometrial cancer among women taking HRT. But it is not a carcinogen. As we know, it simply increases the lining of the womb. But if a cancer is already present, that means the cancer will increase too. And that goes for the breasts as well. However, women who take the combination of oestrogen and progesterone appear to be at no increased risk of developing cancer, compared with women who've been through the menopause and are taking no hormones at all.

The women at highest risk are those who have a family history of endometrial cancer, those suffering hypertension and any one who hasn't carried a baby to full term. Plus women who are massively overweight. About 73 per cent of women who get endometrial cancer are 20 per cent over their healthy body weight.

With **breast cancer** the same risk factors come into play. Obesity doesn't help, and if you suffer from **fibrocystic breast disease** then you are probably already being carefully monitored.

Something else that can be an indicator of breast cancer is if you've had periods for longer than average. If you started your periods before you were twelve, you have four times the risk of developing breast cancer than other women who reach menopause in their mid-forties.

The link between breast cancer and oestrogen usage is still a minefield of debate among doctors. It's a controversial link that many disagree with. Obviously, with the womb, the lining has a chance to be naturally cleared away when stimulated by progesterone. But there's no equivalent dispersal for the breasts. So some women may get abnormal cell growth in the form of benign cysts, and the risk can be increased if these later become malignant and hence cancerous.

Ironically, HRT can actually be of positive benefit in some forms of cancer.

THE PROS AND THE ANTIS

Many medics agree that women who take low dosages of both oestrogen and progesterone run no increased risk of breast cancer.

But then there's the confusing fact that a number of studies have measured an increase in breast cancer among those undergoing oestrogen therapy. It's thought one reason for this is that these women are simply being more closely monitored, so their breast cancers are showing up earlier.

They're screened more often and more thoroughly. And because they're showing up sooner, and perhaps because they're caught earlier, those tumours are often found to be smaller than average. That makes for easier treatment and more likely a complete cure.

So you might wonder why women place themselves at such apparent risk. Why take *any* risk at all? Well, many doctors, and many satisfied customers of HRT, have decided that the benefits far outweigh those risks.

There is the argument, contrary to that of the antis, that women on HRT positively protect themselves against both womb and breast cancer.

The *Journal of the American Medical Association* came out with a study in 1983 on women using HRT and it found they had a lower 'incidence of death of any kind than non-users'. Which means women on HRT were, in the short term, living longer and suffering fewer life-threatening diseases than women who weren't taking it.

Many doctors feel that HRT positively helps the bones and the blood vessels, and prolongs a more active and healthier life.

For a long time it was seen as 'the hair and skin treatment'. But one GP describing changing attitudes to HRT told me, 'It's beginning to be seen less as a "beauty" treatment and more as a medicine these days. However, one has to say there may be long-term effects which we just don't know about. An increasing amount of the news is good, though – unexpectedly good.'

Doctors who are gung-ho about HRT say that unless there are clear and positive indications to avoid HRT, then choosing not to take advantage of it may, in the end, do you more harm than good.

The decision can still be a difficult one. The wealth of information can confuse. We've just been looking at some of the more negative side-effects of HRT. What about the positive ones?

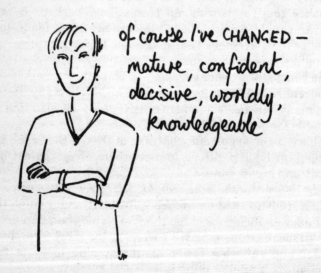

of course I've CHANGED –
mature, confident,
decisive, worldly,
knowledgeable'

CHAPTER 15

The good news

Even the lips stay moist and supple on HRT. It clearly affects all 'soft tissue' areas, not just the vagina. It increases moisture, fullness and elasticity wherever it goes. And that's everywhere. Yes, it may seem to make you younger, but that's only surface value. Father Time marches on and continues to have his slow but inexorable way with the rest of your body, whether you're on HRT or not.

Oestrogen works on the **hair** follicles, so some women notice that their hair gets thicker and shinier than before 'the slide'.

Vaginal dryness is one of the most distressing side-effects of the menopause and usually responds within weeks to treatment. An oestrogen-based cream can be prescribed. That can help too with the vaginal infections that occur more readily after the menopause is over.

In HRT, the slow release of oestrogen and progesterone into the system is also thought to work on the part of the brain called the hypothalamus which affects **mood swings** and **hot flushes**. Here's Jessica's description at age forty-six of her hot flushes, and why she's glad to get rid of them:

'The heat begins in my face and spreads downwards into my neck and chest. Or it reverses and goes the other way. Sometimes I just feel terribly hot all over my body. It only lasts a minute or so. But I find it really disturbing. And then I'm just sitting waiting for the next one. I'm tense and nervous with anticipation. If it's at night, I have to get up and dry myself off with a towel. But then I'm wide awake and can't get back to sleep again.

'Often with a flush I'll get nasty red blotches all over my

face and neck. It's bad enough at night, but really embarrassing in public.

'At the end of the flush I feel cold and strangely weak and fragile. I'm beginning to hate my body and what it does to me. And also, there's something that never happened before: now I seem so full of anxiety about the whole thing that my heart starts beating really hard, and it never did to begin with.'

Combined here are the physical symptoms and the psychological, beginning to weave together a miserable and even frightening series of experiences, which are more unnerving because they are so unpredictable.

Small wonder many women fall on HRT with such relief if it can lessen the discomfort. At the same time as HRT treats hot flushes, it helps other 'vasomotor' symptoms, such as **dizziness**, **palpitations** and **numbness**.

You might also have heard of the endorphin high that runners and athletes get after an energetic workout. It's a natural opiate produced by the body and it's one of the better drugs to be addicted to. Exercise stimulates the release of endorphins. It's thought that levels of these substances rise and fall automatically in sympathy with the oestrogen-progesterone cycle. So lose the cycle, and you lose some of the endorphins too.

BONE FACTS

One of the most important long-term boons of HRT is that it stops the development of **osteoporosis**.

Break down that rather long and ugly word and you can find the syllables 'poros' and that's what it means. Osteoporosis makes the bones more porous.

What is it?
Our bone mass is constantly changing. When we're around eighteen or nineteen, it's at its peak. Then from around thirty to thirty-five we all begin to lose bone at the rate of about 1

per cent a year. As there is less and less calcium in the body, it leaves tiny cavities in the skeleton, like a honeycomb. The bones become spongy, and more brittle. Most of the calcium is simply lost in the urine, but some may accumulate in the bladder or kidney, and stones may form.

Left to its own devices, osteoporosis can eventually become a devastating, crippling disorder which at its best causes pain, and at its worst fractures and deformities.

Who gets it?
It must be said, however, that you can have osteoporosis and never know it. If you don't fall over, or have an accident, or stress any bones too radically, it may never become apparent.

For some people all they have to show for it are the infinitesimal changes in height over the years as the vertebrae gradually compress on each other. It is only if you have the advanced stages of the disease that the vertebrae will actually fracture, causing pain and incapacity.

How many get it?
I've come across different statistics at different times from doctors with different axes to grind. Those who're very pro-HRT say that up to 50 per cent of women are affected by osteoporosis after the menopause. Another figure I came across was that only about 15 per cent of women will get it. Some say 30 to 40 per cent.

The people peddling those numbers may be giving overall figures, but not the *degree* of osteoporosis a woman can experience. Perhaps 50 per cent of women get certain indications of porous bones – but those indications are much less threatening for most than in perhaps the 15 per cent who get it badly.

It's been worked out by the statisticians that about one in four women in this country will suffer from a fracture of some sort in later life. But those are estimates based on an analysis of the old ladies in our population today. Their food intake, medical histories and lifestyles may very well have been altogether different from the women going through menopause now. It may not be possible to genuinely compare the two groups and come to hard and fast results.

Where do you get it?

Osteoporosis can affect any bone. But fractures caused are often related to age. For instance, if they're in their fifties, women are more likely to fracture their wrists. In the sixties, it's the spine that tends to be affected and for the seventy- to eighty-year-olds, it's the hips.

Before hip replacements became more commonplace during the late Seventies, hip fractures alone cost the NHS over £165 million annually. And some twenty thousand women died every year in what came to be called the 'silent epidemic'. About 28 per cent died from the injury. The fall was disabling enough, but it was the pneumonia that followed which often proved fatal.

Forty per cent of all orthopaedic beds were filled with hip fractures and they made up the third largest group of all admissions to hospitals. More women died from osteoporosis and its associated problems than all those who died of cancer of the uterus, cervix and breast put together.

The number of hip fractures in Britain at the moment is running at around fifty thousand a year. In the United States, caring for osteoporosis sufferers costs around six billion dollars annually.

So if you find your doctor waxing long and loud about HRT's ability to *prevent* the condition in the first place, bear with him or her. There's no doubt they're concerned about your health, but they're probably toting up the overall cost to an already overburdened NHS as well.

Why do you get it?

Men get osteoporosis too. But women get it worse. They're smaller than men to start with, so have less skeletal bone mass. After the menopause they can lose bone rapidly, perhaps 2 to 3 per cent a year. By the time she is seventy, a woman may have lost half the bone mass she started out with.

After the menopause, women absorb less calcium from their food and excrete more through the urine. If you have osteoporosis already, and have lost a lot of bone, taking oestrogen will not replace it. It will simply slow down the rate of loss.

Oestrogen helps the body absorb and utilise calcium in the most efficient way. If you don't have enough oestrogen in the body, you will be unable to absorb enough calcium from the food digesting in your gut, no matter how much you eat.

And there are conflicting demands on the calcium we do have. In a strange way, the body goes to war and cannibalises itself, because the blood also needs a constant level of calcium. And if there isn't enough, calcium will be stripped from the bones in order to maintain adequate supplies. The blood gets first call. Your bones get second. And after a long time that will tell on your general health.

The insurance debate
It must be said that not all women are destined to get osteoporosis. You have to decide whether you want to take HRT long-term to prevent something you may never get in the first place.

Battle royal rages between the feminists and drug companies over this issue. The feminists see the debate about osteoporosis as an artificially inflated scare issue. The drug companies, they say, are putting about horror stories implying that all women will suffer this dreadful disease and must take drugs, their drugs, to prevent it.

At the same time it *is* a condition that can ravage old age. 'I don't think women have taken on board what osteoporosis really means,' says a GP who is aware of the problems. 'Unless their mum's broken a hip or they have a string of aunties with it, they don't know how crippling it can be.

'But it's a complicated issue. We're now up to a generation of women who've had thirty years of scares and worry with the Pill. Taking pills for years on end is not the sort of risk-taking behaviour that most women go in for. Most of us will treat the immediate problem. Taking HRT to prevent osteoporosis is a form of insurance. This is an insurance against a risk people haven't identified yet. And that insurance is expensive.'

Who is most at risk?
There are indications you can watch out for to see if you are among those most likely to get it:

★ First, if you've led a **sedentary life**, you are more at risk, because it's well known that exercise stimulates the production of oestrogens, and hence the uptake of calcium. So if you've chosen not to do sport as an adult, or any other systematic physical activity, your body is already at a disadvantage.
★ **Smokers** are at risk. Nicotine inhibits the uptake of calcium, thinning the bones over a long period.
★ Then for some reason that no one has put their finger on, people who are **fair-haired** are also more likely to get osteoporosis.
★ And of course if there's a **family history** of osteoporosis, it's worth having the full check-up.
★ Finally, if you've been pushed into premature menopause because of medical intervention such as a total **hysterectomy**, or because of chemotherapy which has caused **ovarian failure**, many doctors would recommend taking HRT for its protective properties. To suddenly lose the ovaries means an abrupt and complete end of oestrogen production, unlike the more gradual effect of the menopause.

These are all pretty clear indicators. If none of the above applies to you, it means you are more safe than others. You can still get it, but you're certainly at lower risk.

'My worst osteoporosis nightmare patient,' said one GP, 'is the thin, blonde smoker on the tenth floor of a council flat, living on chips.'

The densitometer

Another said the best way of working out who was a long-term risk was to put them on the densitometer machine. Its job is pretty self-evident. It measures your bone density when you first consider going on HRT. That way, you can work out if your bones are already beginning to lose too much calcium.

Needless to say it would be wonderful if every woman could be measured in this way. Then future sufferers would be picked up way ahead of time, treatment could start, and those who don't need to worry could relax. But that scenario is a little Utopian.

Not all the results of present levels of bone density can be confidently and accurately projected, giving absolute forecasts way into the future. We are talking decades here. And this is particularly at a time when they're still experimenting . . .

And more to the point, the problem is there aren't enough densitometers. What's new? Screenings are costly and you'd need five to seven over a six-year period. This particular doctor favoured prescribing HRT for perhaps five or six years, till the menopause was over. Then if the woman showed any indications of being a potential osteoporosis sufferer, she was taken to one of the few densitometers in the health authority and given a screening.

If it's going to work in the prevention of osteoporosis, HRT needs to be taken for ten to fifteen years, or even for life according to some doctors. The downside is that HRT is effective only while you continue to take it. Bones begin to thin again when you stop taking it, and they thin at the same rate as they did before.

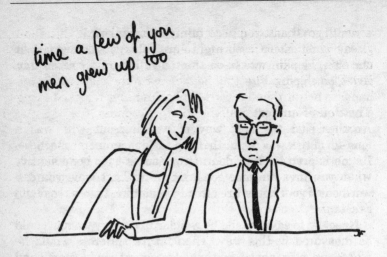

time a few of you men grew up too

AND THERE'S PROTECTION FROM CORONARY HEART DISEASE TOO

A study was done in Framingham, a small city on the east coast of America. This in-depth analysis over thirty years into heart disease found that post-menopausal women who hadn't been taking added oestrogen had more than double the incidence of **coronary heart disease** compared to those who were yet to reach the menopause and still had full supplies of oestrogen circulating in their bodies.

Oestrogen's a little like that lager ad. It reaches the parts that others don't. And in this case, it seems to have a direct and helpful effect on the heart and blood vessel system.

It's been found that women taking oestrogen have less risk of coronary heart disease. Women have always had fewer heart attacks than men. They seem to remain protected for longer. But there does come a time, and it usually coincides with the end of the menopause, when the incidence of heart attack goes up in women and becomes comparable to that of men. But for those women on HRT, their protection seems to stretch for as long as another ten years.

'I went right back to my old figure and my hair is thick and glossy again. Even my breasts – dare I say it – have perked up. And my skin was beginning to go all craggy round my jaw. That's going. Plus that horribly wrinkly "old" look on the hands is better than it was. My husband says it's like having a new me around after all the wimpy tiredness.'
Jean, fifty-two.

'I'm not taking that stuff. Evening Primrose Oil is a godsend. My doctor says I'll come screaming through the door like a banshee when I really need it. But I just don't see it. It's OK. Yes, there are changes. But it feels normal. I'm getting by.'
Mary Rose, forty-nine.

Whatever your choice – an informed consumer is a confident consumer.

CHAPTER 16

Sudden onset or premature menopause

'It was a shock. Just the plain shock of it. It was like a crash course – a helluva bang. I thought it was exhaustion because of "Life" with a capital L but it was the plummeting hormones. And I was still hoping for children. Even though I wasn't in a relationship. But that's been smashed to hell and back. The suddenness somehow felt grotesque. The patch didn't work. Now we're playing around with the pills.'
Fiona, forty.

The mind has almost as much to do with the experience of menopause as the body. If it starts suddenly and early, it can be so much harder to assimilate and adjust to.

In Fiona's case it not only came on suddenly – once there, it all seemed to happen very fast. There was nothing gradual about it. It was abrupt and over practically before it had begun. That was almost more unsettling than anything. A long, slow, gradual decline in hormone production leaves an altogether different slope on the graph than a precipitous fall 'overnight'. Which is how it feels to some women when it happens quickly and unexpectedly.

EARLY MENOPAUSE

If the menopause arrives at the 'usual', expected time, it's easier to be more prepared mentally. There'll be more people around you, going through the same thing, to compare notes with. You'll probably have picked up more information here and there, and generally be more aware of what may be in store.

But for some women, like Fiona, it simply starts a lot earlier than it does for others. Around 5 per cent of women inherit a tendency to early menopause. While they may be surrounded by friends and contemporaries who're still having babies, they themselves are being rushed down the other side of the reproductive hill at an alarming rate.

MENOPAUSE FOLLOWING SURGERY

There are women in their thirties, twenties and sometimes even in their teens who begin the menopause because their ovaries have been destroyed by chemotherapy.

Early menopause can also be brought on if you have to have an operation called an **oöphorectomy**, which means removal of the ovaries and which may be done at the same time as a full **hysterectomy**.

Your own doctor will guide you, but in general, **ovaries** need to be removed to treat ovarian cancer, some oestrogen-dependent cancers of the uterus or breast, severe ovarian cysts and severe endometriosis.

Hysterectomies will be needed to treat endometrial cancers, large uterine fibroids, severe pelvic inflammatory disease, prolapse and excessive uterine bleeding.

A hysterectomy doesn't necessarily involve the removal of the ovaries, though it may if there's something wrong with them as well as with the uterus.

Some surgeons will offer to remove the ovaries at the same time as they do a hysterectomy, even if there's no obvious problem with them. That's because there is a general risk of ovarian cancer for every woman, and perhaps they feel once they're 'in there', they might as well go the whole mile.

Ovarian cancer affects 1 per cent of all women and though you can have regular scans by ultrasound, screening doesn't seem to have had much impact on those death rate figures.

Clearly, when cancers and debilitating gynaecological disorders come into play, removal of uterus or ovaries may be the only route to take.

The downside of having the ovaries taken out is that it trips you straight into menopause – and the virtual inevitability of taking HRT following the op.

Women who for surgical, chemical or natural reasons have an early menopause often need time and attention. Their symptoms can be more severe. If loss of the womb and ovaries is involved, there may be a sadness and grieving.

HYSTERECTOMIES

While on the subject, it's worth noting that we do seem to be moving away from the dark ages. There definitely was a time when it was a fashionable procedure, seen as a cure-all for those apparently intractable 'women's problems'.

Before the importance of oestrogens and progesterones was really understood, there was a definite fashion among doctors to whip out the womb at the slightest opportunity. They would do it for perfectly genuine reasons at the time and it would seem to get rid of the immediate presenting problem.

With hindsight, we can only deduce that for a number of women, it inadvertently created more. And that's especially if the ovaries were removed at the same time as the uterus.

In fact, if you went to America, it would have been wise until very recently to keep your legs crossed and your body as far away from the gynaecologists as possible. Nearly 50 per cent of American women will have hysterectomies at some point in their lives. The op is performed five times more often in the US than on women in Europe. It's a relatively simple procedure surgically and, of course, it's lucrative. American surgeons carry out six hundred and fifty thousand annually. It also has to be said that they carry out operations more often for many other medical conditions as well. But certainly, compared to their European colleagues, they're knife-happy.

Now that we're learning so much more about alternative procedures, those same doctors are admitting that as many as 50 per cent of hysterectomies were unnecessary.

America is notorious for this kind of thing, but we have our own black spots in the UK. It's well recognised that affluent areas where high numbers of women use private medicine have a higher rate of hysterectomies than elsewhere in the country – which is why one sleepy little dormitory town in the South-East has become known in the trade as Wombless Woking.

CHAPTER 17

Linda's story

Linda's story is in many ways a classic. After a long history of medical mismanagement and poor communication, she was lucky enough – in the end – to find the right doctor and the right treatment. She had lived with many years of painful periods and bleeding throughout her menopause.

Like so many life crises, Linda's menopause had seemed to start exactly when she didn't need it. At forty-six years old, she had just moved house for the first time in twenty-five years. As we know, that can feature right at the top of the list of life's stressful events. We've all got our regular daily grumbles, but moving house takes the biscuit on the Geiger stress counter.

She felt that perhaps the upheaval of the move brought on the menopause, but there really is no way of knowing. At the same time, she had a benign growth in her womb removed successfully. So there was a lot going on.

Which is why to begin with, she didn't think too much about her suddenly much heavier and much more painful periods. She put them down to the obvious difficulties of moving, menopause and surgery, all following fast on the heels of each other.

But then she began to realise it was more than that – she really was far more exhausted than she'd ever been. She never had any energy and she was often overwhelmed with a great feeling of lassitude. This from one of those women who can usually do about five different jobs, while spinning on a sixpence and singing 'Dixie'. She had always been full of energy and good health, and it just seemed to drain away.

Her symptoms had started around 1985 and within quick

succession she had two D and Cs. These are minor operations that involve scraping away the lining of the womb, often prescribed for women with heavy bleeding. She had even had, as she called it, some of the 'early' HRT around 1985, when they were still 'finding out about it' and 'it didn't work'.

'Conventional medicine failed me,' is how she describes this time. She went to her new GP with very clear information about what was wrong with her. Linda is one organised woman who sorts out what she is going to say before she says it.

'I was outraged,' she said. 'She (the doctor) wanted to give me Valium. Just like that. At the drop of a hat. Every presenting symptom I had was clearly identifiable as physical. It wasn't depression. It was physiological.'

Sensible though she is, she was so disgusted with her doctor's entirely inappropriate diagnosis and prescription that she stayed away from the medical establishment for three full years. She decided it had nothing for her. Meanwhile her endless tiredness, heavy loss of blood and bad pain went on.

'I was on my knees,' she said when she finally came to the conclusion 'that anything was better than what I was going through.'

So she put her toe back in the waters of mainstream medicine. She changed doctors, and in 1989 went back on to HRT. It's not always easy to change doctors, but if you are really unhappy with the relationship you have with your doc, or the advice you're given, it is a possible option.

It was against her wholistic principles to start taking HRT again, but after a lot of experimentation they eventually got the dose right, unlike the first time.

'The return of energy was amazing. And the mental clarity. It was like a fog lifting.' And that fog, she reckoned, had taken five years out of her life. She feels now that her whole metabolism had slowed down for those full five years.

Then, as life so strangely seems to work out for us, she went through another series of 'challenges', all clustered together. Again she moved – much less stressful. And simultaneously she was promoted at work to head of department. A job demanding time, engagement and energy. All of which she could now provide.

It's a moot point whether she would have got the job in her previous hazy state. The HRT was, she said, 'crucial to her mental health and well-being'.

She started with patches which worked for a year. But she had mild eczema and they began to irritate. So she went on to the pill.

However, through all this, the heavy bleeding had continued, so by 1990 she had her third D and C.

That improved things for a short while, but the pain got worse. In 1991, she was finally referred to a hospital nearby, which luckily for her happened to be a national centre of excellence. It turned out she had an enormous fibroid and some polyps. The doctor said the fibroid had probably been causing the excessive bleeding and increasingly intolerable pain all along.

He also said that with her history, many other places would have simply told her she would have to have a hysterectomy. It's only because they happened to have particularly advanced technology that she didn't. At the time, it was one of the few machines in the country which was able to explore and identify problems deep in the womb.

This is where she marks the turning point in her treatment. Finally, the real problem had been identified. They found out that she had a fibroid, a benign tumour in the uterus, made up of muscle and fibrous tissue embedded in the muscle wall. No one up to this point had known what was wrong with her, either the 'good' GP or the 'bad' GP. And once they discovered it was a fibroid, she was very lucky that this new wonder machine could help them pinpoint the growth's exact location on the uterine wall. That meant they didn't have to take the whole uterus out. They were able to do a relatively simple operation through the vagina, targeting and removing the offending section.

The surgery she had wasn't major. Recuperation was quicker. Thankfully there are more of these machines being used nationally than ever before.

Linda's pain and the heavy bleeding stopped. 'It's so simple,' she said, 'if you've got the knowledge, and equipment and funds . . .'

Linda stayed on HRT until 1993 and then decided she wanted to see if she could come off it. She's had no bleeding at all, apart from a little spotting the first weekend she stopped. But nothing since.

'It's amazing,' she says. 'For the first time in my life I have no bleeding at all.'

She had kept asking, 'When do I stop the HRT?' but no one seemed very clear. None of the health professionals around her knew when the tailing-off period was.

'So, I took it into my own hands, I thought about it very carefully. It's my body and my decision. So why not come off it and see how it goes?' She has a supportive GP now who backs up her right to make her own decisions.

She's had some hot flushes since she's come off, but is weighing up the transient discomfort of those against never having another period in her life. At the moment, she's happy to live with the occasional hot flush. When she was bleeding regularly while on HRT, she often felt tension, and a lack of focus.

'I'm pleased,' she says. 'I think I've gone through the menopause and I don't need to concern myself with HRT any more.'

She does have vaginal dryness. But is, and has been for some time, celibate. She was genuinely surprised at my question because it wasn't something she'd noticed till I brought it up. But yes, come to think of it, she was 'drier' now than when she'd been on HRT.

She's taking Evening Primrose Oil. But more important she's discovered Super Blue-Green Algae. And thinks she might be on to something.

Algae rank among the first ever life forms found on the

planet. In their simple cell-like structures, then and now, can be found the basic blue-print for the multitude of life forms that followed. The first link in the food chain, made when sunlight plays on water, they are even more basic to biological life than bacteria. For billions of years they have dwelt in every drop of water and every inch of fertile soil, transforming minerals, gases and sunlight into food for plant and animal life.

Algae can be grown commercially and harvested in algae ponds, a bit like salmon farms. Some types are foraged wild. Algae are made edible by a drying-out process and are rich in Vitamin B12 plus many minerals and trace elements.

Super Blue-Green Algae grow naturally in the volcanic, clear, mineral-rich waters of Lake Oregon. Blue-Green promise increased vitality, mental clarity, and relief from sluggishness and fatigue.

At time of writing Linda is fifty-four. She's only been taking Blue-Green Algae for four months since she's stopped HRT, but she swears by them.

She feels good. She's had no massive withdrawal symptoms. She's physically fit.

It doesn't really matter what you take – as long as it works for you. If Blue-Green Algae work, take them. If you prefer HRT – take that.

What's important is to know that there are choices. It's only by experimenting and passing word down the grapevine that we can learn what works for some women and what works for others. Revamping a lifestyle in mid-life can be challenging. It's good to know there are options.

It's also good to know that one of the proven options for easing many an ache and pain during the change is sex.

CHAPTER 18

Sexual healing –
how to hitch a ride
on the happy hormone

'The difference between then and now is that now I know it's going to be great and I don't even think about coming. I don't know when I stopped worrying. Sometime during my menopause.'
Vera, fifty-four.

'The walls of my vagina are much thinner than they ever used to be. But during sex they plump up again, firmer than they ever used to. And they stay firm too – for quite a while.'
Hilda, sixty-four.

'Sex? I didn't know I was *born* till after my menopause. It changed everything.'
Rachel, fifty-five.

'Suddenly all that contraceptive stuff was gone. There's just no thought about getting pregnant. You knew even in those days you wouldn't get pregnant because you were doing something about it. But it was always on your mind. Now I don't have to think about it at all. It frees it all up somehow. We're getting down to the real business at hand. There's only one focus. Pleasure.'
Beth, fifty-three.

'I've always loved sex. What's the menopause got to do with it?'
Liz, forty-eight.

'In the absence of anything else – and that's quite a lot of the time – I use the vibrator. What a godsend.'
Su, forty-eight.

'Sex is the same. It doesn't change. Yet it's different too. It's more fulfilling.'
Catherine, fifty-one.

'I was dry as a bone. It hurt during sex. It hurt after sex. Especially peeing. For a long time after. Then I divorced my husband. Now I just have to see my new lover across the room and I can feel the wet oozing out.'
June, thirty-seven.

'I didn't like it. I didn't want it. But you can't hold back the clock. Menopause comes to us all. And then the strangest thing happened. Something clicked. Suddenly I realised in a way I never had before, time was running out. And it's precious. I only discovered my clitoris six years ago. Now I

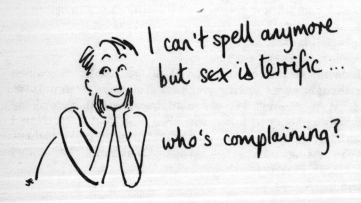

I can't spell anymore but sex is terrific ... who's complaining?

don't wait for them to find it. I tell them where it is. And what to do with it.'
Susan, forty-nine.

'Massage! That's my latest thing. Try it. It's so great. I can't believe what I've been missing. It's the soft, smooth hands all over my body for ages. And then concentrating on my genitals last. I've never had sex like it.'
Jen, fifty-three.

'I hate that phrase, "use it or lose it". It's so peremptory. So bossy. But it's true.'
André, fifty-six.

'After sex it was always me who got the bottle of wine. Or refilled the glasses. Or fetched a snack and put the music on again. Fuck that. Now he does it. It's taken me half a lifetime to get there.'
Jennifer, fifty.

'I used to hold in all this passion I felt. It was so wild. So enormous. I thought it might frighten them. Now I just let rip. I don't care anymore. It's there. And it's great.'
Muna, forty-nine.

'They've changed over the years. When I was in my twenties my orgasms were urgent and quick. Then in my thirties they were more intense and longer. Then they kind of slowed even more and became more gentle. But now they're really deep and penetrating and long. But then so are my fantasies lately. You learn a thing or two over time. It makes all the difference.'
Jessica, fifty-seven.

'He gets his. Why shouldn't I do what it takes to get mine? And believe me, I do.'
Meg, forty-six.

'If they don't want to know my clitoris, I don't want to know them.'
Fiona, fifty-two.

'We must both have been having these fantasies for years. Wrapped up in our own different worlds. But now we've started talking about them and acting them out. It's incredible. What took us so long?'
Pat, sixty-two.

'Now I want it and he doesn't.'
Sandra, fifty-six.

'Everyone bangs on about lubrication. But I'm post-menopausal. I'm not on HRT. And I'm juicy. The trick in staying sexy is to keep having sex. Good sex, that is.'
Michelle, fifty.

'Of course I want a relationship. But I'd rather have nothing than go through what I went through before. Somehow these days I'm more prepared to put me and my needs first. Now I know what they really are.'
Laurie, forty-seven.

'I can't believe it. I never used to *ask* before. Now I do. I make it clear as day what I want. And I come every time.'
Kit, fifty-one.

'If I don't have regular sex, I put weight on.'
Maria, fifty-three.

CHAPTER 19

Love is a drug –
don't kick the habit

Simone de Beauvoir tells a wonderful story of talking to a woman of eighty and asking her when an old lady becomes incapable of sex. 'I don't know,' she said. 'You'll have to ask someone older than me.'

Amazed though some youngsters might be at what their elders and betters are getting up to, the truth of the matter is that a recent survey showed that 91 per cent of people over sixty still have regular sex – retired couples on average one and a half times a week.

Sex releases the happy hormones, endorphins, which not only make you feel good, they do you good. They bathe you in a glow of well-being. Scientists have measured the chemical changes in the brain after sex and say the endorphins work much like alcohol, remaining in the system for hours afterwards.

But instead of a hangover that wipes us out the next morning, they linger gently, reducing tension and irritability. Orgasm brings a physical release that is one of the best stress busters in the business. Get rid of stress and the relaxation that automatically follows has been credited as one of the greatest cure-alls, from easing migraines to helping to fend off colds and flu, and generally boosting the immune system.

SEX AND THE MENOPAUSE

If menopause is a subject still clothed in silence – sex and the menopause is wrapped in even darker veils. Body and mind can go through sweeping changes during 'the change'. And at the very heart of that complex web of experience lies the most sensitive and intimate area of all – a woman's attitude to her sexuality. Whatever the nature and quality of her sex life, some of the greatest reassessments and changes that occur during the period of the menopause can be to do with sex and sensuality.

There has always been a faintly curious attitude to sex and older people. Back in the relative dark ages of the last century, women who wanted sex 'after a certain age' were said to be driven by 'morbid impulses'.

The medics went so far as to say that the post-menopausal woman who 'indulged' could experience excessive bleeding, cancers of the womb, even insanity. A woman marrying late in life was considered wise if she went to her doctor for advice first.

Some residual prejudices still lurk. They are less obviously noxious, but they can still colour social attitudes. They can also cling with surprising force. Many we carry without being aware – such as that of the post-menopausal woman as a dried-up old stick or the older woman as sexually neutered.

Even so, things are better. Thankfully we have crawled out from under the stone of that late nineteenth century paranoia. It's clear from the women's comments in the last chapter that even if some public attitudes are skewed, on a personal level sex offers a rich and abundant wealth of experience, either as an ongoing re-affirmation of a deep and satisfactory long-term relationship, or as a voyage of discovery into new and unknown delights.

All the women quoted, except June who's thirty-seven, are talking about sex and the menopause. For many, their sex lives changed – and for the better.

Some women continue to have active and happy sex lives before, during and after the menopause. For them there is no disruption. Others are not so lucky and the changes they're going through, mentally and physically, leave them less willing or even able to keep having sex with their partners.

We often hear more about the latter because they're the ones doctors are concerned about. More information is written about and for them. After all, if you've just got out of bed after a night of quadruple orgasms with the earth moving on the hour every hour, you are not likely to go to your doctor to get things fixed. They aren't broke.

There's a myth circulating that women at the menopause either turn off sex completely, or become voracious, raging sex-fiends. The ones who have difficulty may have always had difficulty, but at the menopause decide to throw in the towel and stop trying:

'I put up with it for years. But I always promised myself when I got to the menopause that that's when I'd stop his fiddling around. I'm past putting up with it.'
Eva, fifty-three.

THE MENOPAUSE AND SEXUAL LIBERATION

Self-image changes at this time. Until the new post-menopausal woman emerges from her chrysalis, some women become unsure of themselves and their attractiveness, and that can include sexual attraction too.

We live in a world where men who put it about are called studs. Women who are identified as wanting it 'often' (how often is often?) are called nymphomaniacs. With such double standards in operation, it's almost impossible to really get an objective measurement of female desire. But there is no doubt that something significant can and does happen to many women at the menopause which seems to liberate and release them sexually in a way that they haven't been before. Sex is better. And because it is better they do want more.

What fascinates about those personal vignettes is how they reflect the different sexual experiences of different generations. Again and again I hear older women talk of the sheer relief of never having to worry about contraception again.

I'm sure that's the case for all women as they finally climb off that reproductive wheel. Indeed, most post-menopausal women clearly state it. But for the women whose sex life started pre-Pill, I've noticed an even keener relief. Their sexuality was shaped at a time when contraception was more complicated. The climate was more sexually repressed. The release is even greater.

Something else you can tease out from the different individual stories is the shift in the power play between the sexes, and how this can radically change a woman's intimate experience with her partner. That too can be coloured by the decade when she came to sexual maturity. Each generation has its different markers.

I wonder if the young women of today with a lifetime of supposed sexual emancipation behind them, will get the same sense of liberation when they reach their menopause?

POWER PLAY

I have a very vivid memory of a conversation I had over ten years ago, with a woman of about sixty-five. It was at one of those gatherings you have at Christmas in a neighbour's house. It's only at those big bashes that you get such a fertile cross-section of generations. She was a lovely, gentle woman and very interested in my life and my work and what I was doing. But her last words sent a chill through me. She heard all my hopes and plans, and then remarked how lucky I was to have my own life. 'It wasn't like that for us. In my day, dear, we had to please our husbands.'

I don't for one moment think she was talking about pleasing her husband in bed. And yet the bottom line of the deal she had to strike was that to secure an economically secure base for herself and her children, over and above all things, including her own needs, she had to please her husband. The power play was unequal.

To a greater or lesser extent, something happens to many

women at menopause that liberates them from that bind. These days things are supposed to be more equal. And indeed socially and economically they are. There are not the same constraints as there once were. Times have changed. We have more choices about staying in, or leaving relationships.

But the power play doesn't go away. It just moves into different territory. And what a lot of menopausal women seem to be saying is – 'For so long I've done it this way. Well, that doesn't work for me any more. Now I'm going to do it *that* way.' Suddenly they just don't care about the implications any more. And from that comes a great liberation. Particularly in bed.

Funnily enough, going back to Eve who didn't want her husband 'fiddling round with her any more', all she was doing was stating her preferences and acting on them. It can cut both ways. She had always felt them, yet had only managed to give voice to them when she reached the menopause. Somehow, arriving at that certain time of life conferred a new status with new 'rights' – and she was going to invoke them.

CHANGING YOUR ATTITUDES

'The change' really does mean change. Even for those who're immediate descendants of the sexual revolution.

The continuous thread woven through all the conversations I had was that something shifted in the attitudes of those women to their own needs. They were now putting those needs first. The fall-out can be far-reaching. Many had lived a lifetime of caring and nurturing and supporting others. Now it is time for them. There is a re-orientation. But it's something they have to generate for themselves because no one else will.

Older women's sexuality is a secret garden more dense and unexplored than most. Even Shere Hite's ground-breaking book, *The Hite Report*, exploring women's sex lives, devotes only fourteen out of four hundred and thirty-eight pages to older women.

Menopause can catapult a woman into reassessing much about her life, not least how she feels about her own body. At the same time comes a more pressing realisation that time flies. Life is passing by and unless you grab it with both hands it'll slip through your fingers like dry sand.

This potent cocktail can galvanise as nothing has before. Which is when you get the women who, though they change nothing outwardly in their lives, seem to have a new, deeper purpose and clarity about where they're going and why. Or you get the women who suddenly take off and for the first time in their lives they're game for everything. The 'try anything once' brigade.

They are liberated by a new view of themselves. They've got substantial life experience to draw on. They know more surely than ever before what will and will not work for them. And that never holds more true than of what they want and need from a partner sexually. It can be a powerful stimulant. One that can bring even greater satisfaction to both.

So shifting attitudes of mind play a powerful role at this time. But meanwhile, we still have the body to deal with.

GETTING PHYSICAL

There are women who have very real physical discomfort which for the first time affects the pleasure of both them and their partners. This can be fixed.

For some it's the purely mechanical problem of a vagina which doesn't lubricate as well or as readily as before. As with hot flushes, not all women experience this symptom. And it can be something that comes and goes. But when it's there, there's no denying it, and it needs attention.

This for many is one of the worst of the menopausal

symptoms. **Vaginal dryness** is uncomfortable. But its current bad press may be a throw-back to when women were embarrassed to talk about it, and suffered unnecessarily and for too long. If one is going to feel faintly shamed and degraded about the menopause, there is something about this particular symptom that seems to capture all that is negative.

Yet the discomfort can be so quickly solved. Treatments available which I have already mentioned are oestrogen creams and water-soluble K-Y Jelly, which can help enormously.

But one of the best prescriptions for it is regular sex. As far back as the Sixties, Masters and Johnson were recommending increased sexual activity for menopausal women. Older women needed more sex, they said, than their younger counterparts – to keep the glands in working order by keeping them working.

Climaxing regularly can specifically help with other vaginal problems too. One of the recurring symptoms at the end of the menopause can be **thrush**. It's thought that thrush may develop sometimes if a woman is sexually aroused, but doesn't reach orgasm, which is something that can happen to the menopausal woman. Anything from physical symptoms to poor self-esteem can lead to a temporary halt in a woman's sex life. But that doesn't mean she isn't at times aroused. She may remain sensually expectant, but sex for her isn't consummated by an orgasm.

Sensual arousal increases blood levels in the pelvic region, changing the pH or acidity levels. That raises the temperature in the vagina. On orgasm, that congestion is released. But if you don't climax it remains, and harmful yeast organisms have an ideal breeding ground.

But even if you have a regular and satisfying love life, sex itself may still not be happening often enough to maintain the same balance that there was before oestrogen levels started falling. Or perhaps you may not be in a relationship at present, so regular sex can't be relied on.

DO-IT-YOURSELF

In the long list of women's experiences at the beginning of the last chapter, I deliberately included June because although she wasn't menopausal she did have one of the classic menopausal symptoms, **vaginal dryness**.

Dry vaginas can develop at any time in your life. In her case the cure was divorce and a new lover. A shake-up as radical as this is not for everyone. Luckily for her, as soon as her life circumstances changed so did her 'problem'. But not all of us would want that kind of upheaval. There are other ways to get those mucous glands going.

If you go to your doctor and complain of a dry vagina, s/he is more likely to prescribe you HRT than masturbation. But there are those who say the second will do you just as much good.

Orgasm is simply a way of engorging the vagina with blood – keeping the tissues healthy and fed. An orgasm two or three times a week will keep the secretions flowing. Plus the contractions will exercise the womb and the vagina. Women who are aroused and have full intercourse, but don't reach orgasm do not get the benefits of the engorgement of blood that follows from the rhythmic muscle spasm of full release and satisfaction. Sex has to ring that bell to have the full effect.

Some women have warm and loving partnerships which don't lead to sex that often. Some women don't have partnerships and actively chose to remain celibate. Many sensibly continue to masturbate throughout and after menopause, not just for pleasure, but for good health.

Shere Hite questioned over three thousand women for her *Report*. Their ages ranged from fourteen to seventy-eight. Eighty-two per cent said they masturbated and 'could orgasm easily and regularly whenever they wanted'.

Which doesn't mean that it doesn't still have guilt and repression attached. Masturbation doesn't exactly rank high in most topics of conversation. One woman reported being beaten when 'caught' masturbating at eight. She was told she would go mad. She didn't touch her clitoris again till she was forty-six. And even then, with trepidation.

Many women with dry vaginas don't really notice, unless they suddenly have sex after a long absence. Some women however have discomfort simply from everyday friction.

We put oil in our cars to keep them going. Are our cars really more important than our sex lives? Let's not forget the fine example set by the Georgian Abkhazians, the Kashmiri Hunzas and the Colombian Vilcambas who went on having regular sex well into their nineties.

Masturbation has a venerable tradition. There are sculptures of dildos from Babylonian and Indian art from thousands of years ago. In China the women of the aristocracy would indulge their sexual desires using a couple of golden balls. A small one was inserted into the vagina, then a second one after that to act as a bulwark at the entrance. The small ball would roll back and forwards along the vaginal cavity, kept in place by the bigger. The women would then clamber on to swings and swing back and forwards until they'd had their wicked way with themselves.

At one point Masters and Johnson became worried about the use of dildos, saying women were becoming addicted to them. Holy Moly!

Shere Hite is interesting when talking about the way that women's sexuality is analysed. Sexual intercourse with a partner is assumed to be the basic expression of female sexuality. All research questions proceed from that assumption. How about letting the women set the agenda she says, and instead of telling them what they should feel, ask them what they *do* feel?

For many, masturbation is far from second-rate sex.

Frequent orgasm, however it happens, is good for you. It lowers the cholesterol in your blood. It increases the amount of fat-burning hormones released into the system, and it gives you exercise in the nicest possible way. The exertion pushes the pulse, blood pressure and respiration levels up to those of professional athletes. Muscles contract all over the body, voluntarily and involuntarily, from head to toe. For anyone who's counting, you burn up two hundred calories over a fifteen-minute spell of active sex.

Perhaps GPs should think again about those prescriptions.

HELP YOURSELF

With age, the lining of the vagina becomes thinner. The texture of the skin changes too. It gets smoother, with fewer ridges and small bumps, and it changes from the deep rose pink of its youth to a lighter shade. Its length and width reduce too. But again, with regular use, it can remain just as elastic with the same capacity it has always had. Women still have contractions of the womb on orgasm when past the menopause. And their nipples and clitoris still broaden in diameter and become erect on stimulation.

The amount of your vaginal secretion is probably going to depend on the amount of lust you feel for your partner, or the potency of your sexual fantasy. But the 'juices' come from the Bartholin's glands which lie right behind the entrance to the vagina. They can be stimulated by fantasy, touch and scent. For example, **aromatherapy** oils.

Aromatherapists have been successfully treating women with the problem of vaginal dryness for years. You can make up your own massage formula from any of the following quintessential oils. But a session or two with an aromatherapist could come in handy, just to see which combinations, in which quantities, work best for you.

The oils which help lack of vaginal secretion are: geranium, sandalwood, hyacinth, cinnamon, rose bulgar, ylang-ylang, lavender, nutmeg, clary, neroli, savory, benzoin, vervain, cypress, anis and fennel.

Make up your own formulas to your own taste, or rather smell, adding them in combinations to good (unscented) skin oils which you can get in health shops. Ten drops each of geranium, lavender and fennel go well together. Or try fifteen drops of sandalwood, five drops of neroli and four of vervain. Cypress, hyacinth and clary work well. Massage them on to your lower abdomen, breasts and the small of the back. Add them to your bath. Rose bulgar is particularly luxurious. Or a combination of scents works too.

Rose bulgar goes well with geranium and vervain. Geranium, lavender and fennel are a delight, both as a bath combination as well as for massage. Rose bulgar, also known as maroc, can mix happily with clary, fennel and hyacinth.

Use the oils in daily baths for a week, as well as combining the scents in a massage mix – again on a daily basis. Some women report lubrication returning and penetration getting easier within three days.

Taking time to nurture your own needs can be one of the positive benefits of the new-found assurance that comes at this time.

One woman told of how she liked to be covered all over in cream because she enjoyed the enormous sensuality of her

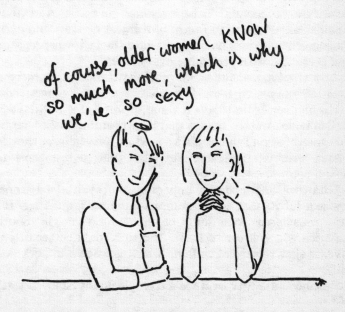

of course, older women KNOW so much more, which is why we're so sexy

lover licking it off. Another talks of taking a whole day to plan a candlelit dinner followed by sex, the excitement beginning when she wrote out the shopping list in the morning. The anticipation of the climax to come began as she listed all the luscious things to buy for that evening. By the time she'd got to putting on the silk underwear and dimming the lights, she could barely contain herself.

Aphrodisiacs can be fun to play with. The giggle factor is probably as erotic as the substances themselves. They've been used since time began to loosen lust. And there's no time like the present to see if they work for you.

Hand round the bread basket at a Roman feast and you were likely to have an orgy on your hands before you could say Dance of the Seven Veils. The Romans used to knead aphrodisiacs into their bread rolls and use them as a little light aperitif that did more than perk up the taste buds.

Quite what the ingredients were it's hard to know. Different cocktails and concoctions have been used down through the ages. In all up to nine hundred substances have been identified as having lust-provoking qualities. And that includes asses' testes in broth, bird intestine stew and even the penis of wolves. Though quite how the last was prepared and presented we'll probably never know.

Just thinking about some of those things is more of a turn-off, than a turn-on. But there are many other foods, herbs and spices that have a venerable pedigree in the Food Hall of Love. And the reason they do is that they either mimic the smell of sexual chemicals we produce naturally, or they're loaded with vitamins and nutrients that give a boost to sexual pep.

Guaraná has made an impact on the health-food scene. It's sold for its fast-acting stamina-enhancing qualities. It's also considered something of an aphrodisiac in South America where it comes from. And that could be because it gives a slow release of caffeine which is known to perk you up.

Casanova ate fifty **oysters** a day. No doubt he loved their slimey yukkiness. But as well as the sensuous pleasure he got from letting them slither down his throat, he was also delivering a massive dose of zinc into his system. Oysters are packed with zinc which has a similar effect to that of the natural chemical, histamine. **Histamine** helps ejaculation in men and, apparently, increases the libido in women.

Any substance that works on smell can be particularly powerful. Our sense of smell takes stimulants straight through delicate membranes direct to the brain. Saliva, genital secretions and sweat all contain pheromones. No one knows quite how they work, except that they stimulate the brain's sex centre. And quickly. Anything that reminds you of those three smells and juices excites the brain and could excite you.

It'll take some ingenuity, but if you can think of a recipe that combines garlic, anchovies, wheatgerm and honey, you'll be rocking the night away.

Garlic scores high. Given its anti-social connotations, it's hard to believe that at the height of our sexual pleasure, we give off a smell similar to that of this humble little onion. So its associations stimulate memories of good vibrations.

Anchovies are laden with phosphorus, good for sexual function. **Wheatgerm** is one of the richest available sources of Vitamin E, the 'fertility' vitamin. And **honey** gives energy.

Both **truffles** and **parsley** imitate the musky male hormone, androsterone. You might think it's his sense of humour that turns you on, but it could be his close resemblance to a herb garden. One hundred grammes of fresh white truffles were selling for £160 at the last count, so plump for the parsley. It's probably just as good.

You can literally spice up your love life with a sexy scorcher of **ginger**, **pepper**, **nutmeg** and **cayenne**. They're all stimulants, and will work on the whole body. And **caraway** has been used in love potions since the times of Ancient Egypt.

Enjoy.

CHAPTER 20

Is it all in the genes?

The menopause is so broad. Women's experience can be so random. Without rhyme or reason one woman has it good, while another has a long, hard haul. So much seems to be down to luck. And the rest is down to genetics – what's been inherited from parents.

There are those lucky women who seem to have untroubled gynaecological histories. Puberty arrives quietly. They ovulate, menstruate, conceive and bear children in the alloted time-span given them, and then they go through a gradual menopause with a tweak and a twinge here and there, but nothing to get too worried about.

For others, it's a different story. Some women have a genuinely poor time. And many feel isolated and alone. They reach the end of their tether before seeking help and then are amazed that there are people who will not only listen, but who also seem to understand. 'I didn't know other women went through this too,' they say.

We've come a long way. The menopause debate is out there on the public agenda more clearly than ever before. But even yet, we can improve things. Because there are still women who are suffering in silence. And that suffering is unnecessary.

We can do a lot ourselves to ease the load.

THE SUB-PLOT

First of all, let's get back to basics and tease out the cluster of attitudes that surround the menopause.

The main anxiety underpinning the whole thing, whether it's good or bad, is that the menopause is tangible proof that you are ageing.

It's time to chuck that out the window. Once and for all, let's debunk the myth that the menopause itself makes people old. You age from the moment you are born.

The lens of the eye becomes less elastic from early childhood. Eyesight can be past its peak by adolescence. Collagen, which makes up a third of our total body protein, becomes increasingly tough and less flexible. The years between thirty and fifty see the most rapid changes in women *and men*.

Nerve-muscle coordination slows down, in both sexes, from thirty onwards. Movements are less precise. Elasticity begins to go. Muscles shrink, especially the ones we don't exercise. Hair thins. From about forty to forty-five, both sexes become long-sighted and start having difficulties hearing high-pitched tones. Organ function slows down. The metabolism loses speed. *Both* sexes, to a greater or lesser extent, get heart disease, arterial disease, hypertension, arthritis, rheumatism and other 'age'-related syndromes.

Before you put the gun to your temple – there is hope. First, both sexes age in roughly the same way at roughly the same rates. The menopause does not cause ageing. It is not part of the ageing process. It is something programmed into us from conception.

Ageing is natural. It is simply the mark of the passage of time. We can do so much to change those blows into gentle brush strokes – if not banish them from our lives for many a year.

Yet still we panic. We might know all of the above intellectually. But fear of ageing is rooted deep. Menopause is such a concrete physical experience. It carves its notch on our lives so markedly that we overload it with all the charged and negative emotion associated with fear of death.

Bags, sags and wrinkles take on a more significant meaning, even if they've been hanging around for years. They suddenly give off a signal that is undeniable. A threshold has been reached. A step forward is inevitable. A door is closing behind us.

And that's unnerving. Some people swear they don't mind, and seem to carry it off with grace and serenity. And indeed many women do get a new surge of energy and meaning at this time of life. Jobs change for the better. Marriages and partnerships re-focus and find new layers of communication. Relationships with children reassemble into adult coalitions. The sky is bluer. The sun shines.

But for the rest of us, it's not unlikely that for a transition time at least, we may be all of a twitch. Symptoms will be ignored. And we'll turn a blind eye to the obvious, until finally suppression doesn't work any more.

Suddenly, there we are. Past even that age when you start being grown up. Yes, we are at last, without doubt, middle-aged.

But 'middle-aged' is such an irritatingly loose and woolly measurement. In the old days, the 'middle-aged woman' did self-effacing good works and played the dutiful wife waiting with carpet slippers and pipe. But no longer. More and more women, particularly with current levels of unemployment, are sole breadwinners. And if not that, they're committed to work and a degree of independence unheard of in their mothers' time.

These days we can expect better health into old age. The quality of life has improved and as these women look forwards to the one whole third of the life that remains before them – they're demanding more. Social, economic and cultural oblivion is now no longer acceptable. Soon the pensionable age will be equal, a move welcomed by many women who want to remain engaged in the world outside their home.

Even as we speak, older women are forging a new path for themselves. And the tracks they lay down will have a direct bearing on the route the rest of us take as we follow.

One of the first steps down that road is to reject and dismiss the clichés about shrivelled up ovaries and old bags who're past it once they're menopausal.

It's a pernicious slight used as a weapon of oppression. It's only as hundreds of thousands, even millions, of older women live out their vital, healthy and fulfilled lives that we'll ever prove that it's an ideology rooted in ignorance and fear.

These days, scientists experimenting in laboratories have been able to double an animal's lifespan. As they understand more and more about cell structure, they're coming up with ideas for the slowing down of the march of time. But so what? The need to search for eternal youth, or perhaps eternal life, seems to be carved through our genes. However, it's a pointless fantasy that isn't worth a tuppenny farthing if we're not going to get the quality of that life right.

Age barriers are tumbling. The old order is being challenged. Expectations will continue to rise. The decisions a menopausal woman takes at this junction will radically determine the quality of her health for the rest of her days. But as she gingerly picks her solitary path through this new order, it's worth remembering that these days the sky's the limit.

HOLDING BACK THE YEARS

Father Time is not the ogre he was. There are more older people living now than ever before. We're living longer and with better health. Even political clout will begin to shift as the 'grey panthers', currently misnamed 'old-age pensioners', carry a larger percentage of the vote and start stalking the corridors of power. By the year 2010, there'll be more people over sixty than under.

That is going to force changes in current social trends and attitudes. But where is the individual in all of this? We will still be ageing. But how? The political does become personal. These days we're learning more and more about the physical aspects of ageing. Take it on board at your menopause, or even before, and you'll sail through those golden years.

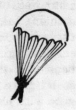

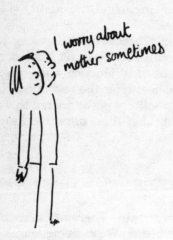

I worry about
mother sometimes

VIRTUAL SHANGRI-LA

We've all heard about extraordinary countries where people
live to one hundred and twenty. They always come from
somewhere romantically remote, live on an impossibly
restricted diet, and work the fields from dawn till dusk.

I don't know why they don't turn the whole of central
Abkhazia in Soviet Georgia into a twenty-first century New
Age laboratory. The people there have no tooth decay, no

heart disease, no mental illness, no obesity, no cancer. Alexander Leaf from Harvard Medical School spent several years studying them, as well as the Vilcamba Indians in the Andes, and the Hunzas in mountainous Kashmir.

He chose them for the simple reason that they were all known to live very long lives, some supposedly up to one hundred and forty years.

So what do they have in common? Do they brew potent bevvies from secret ingredients laced with liquids from subterranean tracts hidden in deepest caverns? Do they offer up mesmerising incantations to a god of time inaccessible to the rest of us?

No. They simply lead extremely active lives. Even the ninety-year-olds spend many hours a day working hard in the fields, or on the mountainsides. They all have a very low-calorie diet. We eat around 3,000 to 3,500 calories a day. They get by on around 1,700. And of that 1,700 calories, there is little fat or animal protein; most sustenance comes in the form of raw, fresh vegetables, rough grains and fruit. They've never heard of sugar. Their vegetables are organic, free of artificial fertilisers.

Then there's the sex. They were all leading very active lives physically anyway, but sex continued well into their eighties and nineties.

It's unlikely that many of us will ever spend six or seven hours a day ploughing, reaping and winnowing. We're never going to toil in the fields. The farmers wouldn't let us on their land. They've got machines to do the job. The human body as provider of brute force is redundant.

Which leaves us to our own devices.

CHAPTER 21

It don't mean a thing
if it ain't got that zing

Zest for life is within the reach of everyone. Extra vitality and stamina can transform a routine day into something that bit special. Some people seem to be born with energy in abundance. But the rest of us can do a lot to top up those natural supplies.

So far we've looked at the physical aspects of the menopause. Next, it's self-help. What we can do for ourselves. The choices open to us. The decisions we can take. How we can make a substantial impact on the quality of our lives.

The menopause is a bridge to the last third of our lives. It is not too late to lay plans and have dreams. And it's not too late to make changes. Whatever the route you take – better to be in the driving seat than travel as a passenger.

The medical world offers enormous relief. But we can treat ourselves too. Treat ourselves with food, with exercise, with fun. And as important, treat ourselves with luxuries. There's so much that's just there for the taking.

I can remember when filming a health series called *Well-Being* over a decade ago that we got terribly excited because we were able to report about the first Health Corner that Sainsbury's had installed as an experiment, 'to see if people were interested or not'.

Interested? The health boom has rocketed. The idea now of a Health Corner seems faintly quaint. It's had its day. And that's because the products in health corners and health shops have percolated into the mainstream. As have the philosophies behind them. And that's only to the good.

There's more information freely available than ever before about food, exercise, health, and the many ways of increasing our stamina and boosting energy levels.

More and more of us check for unnecessary sugars and salts on the labels of the food we buy. Organic vegetables are appearing on ordinary supermarket shelves. Safeway stock over two hundred organic foods in their three hundred and fifty stores nationwide. The only reason they stock them is that they can make money from them. Sainsbury's very own home-grown organic Little Gem lettuce has won prizes at the National Organic Food Awards. Consumers are voting with their taste-buds. It's heartening to know, as we trawl our trolleys round those monster mansions of food retailing, that we do have power.

Where exercise is concerned, you're no longer a loony if you go jogging. And believe me, when I was working on the Channel 4 health series *Well-Being*, which wasn't that long ago, anyone who broke into a sweat because they voluntarily took exercise had some explaining to do. The explosion of knowledge about well-being has been enormous.

Not least in the field of the menopause. We know more. We talk about it more. Treatments continue to get more effective.

But even so, much of what we experience and the way in which we're treated is dependent on us dealing with the medics and 'experts'. It can be alarming at the onset of menopause to have to adjust to 'the change'. And it's good to get as much help as necessary. And essential, of course, if the symptoms are physically intolerable or even life-threatening.

But what we're looking at now is how we can *self*-treat. What's on the market. What's available. What's the latest buzz.

CHAPTER 22

It don't mean a thing
if you can't shake and swing

'Exercise! Never! I know it's good for me but . . . um . . .'

'I've joined a new club and I'm *definitely* going to go to some classes this time.'

'. . . so after Christmas it became a hatstand, though it *was* thoughtful of her to give me an exercise bike.'

'I would go but my work/partner/baby/motor maintenance classes/chores/stamp collection/cat take up too much of my time already.'

If the Vilcambas, Hunzas and Abkhazians can do it at ninety, so can we.

'Exercise is the single most significant thing you can do to break old patterns and start anew,' said a nutritionist I spoke to. You'd think she'd talk about food first. But she said, 'Get the exercise right and the body gets fitter. You feel better. As soon as you feel better, you eat better. Automatically.'

It doesn't matter what you do, but it's worth considering doing *something* – anything. Run. Jog. Swim. Rebound. Box. Do aerobics. Do yoga. Cycle. Go to the gym. Walk. Skip. Row. Jazz dance. Tap dance. Belly dance. Do whatever you feel you'll enjoy most. Maybe a combination of a few things so that boredom doesn't settle in. If you don't exercise already, it will change your life.

Get that heart rate up. Get those lungs working. Regular exercise will increase your energy. It won't tire you out. Taking time out of your life to get fit will put more time back into your life in increased vitality and concentration.

There's a wonderful powerhouse of energy in every cell in our body. It's packed into the section called the mitochondria. When you lift your little finger, or a thought passes across your mind, or you produce a hormone, digest a carrot, or get on a running machine – your body draws energy from this source.

Six months after you start exercising regularly, big chances begin to take place in your cells. The number of mitochondria increase. There are more sites producing more energy.

So if you feel low in energy and daunted by the prospect of any exercise at all, take heart. It won't deplete you even more. For the first time in your life you'll be producing excess energy. Menopausal women often suffer a drop in energy. This could be one way to get some back.

It's no good sitting on the sofa watching Linford Christie run the fastest one hundred metres in the world and thinking, 'I can't do that, I might as well give up.' Luckily no one will be measuring your performance for the foreseeable future. Anyone around you is probably too busy panting and puffing, just aiming for their own personal targets.

IT'S BEEN PROVED

Exercise can make you more emotionally stable, self-sufficient, imaginative and confident. Exercise enough and you can develop greater mental acuity, concentration and willpower.

Purdue University in the United States carried out a study on some middle-aged people who didn't exercise and had sedentary jobs. They volunteered for a four-month fitness programme with psychological tests before and after. All of them were put through what's called the 'Cattel Sixteen Personality Factor Questionnaire'. The exercise they had to do was mainly running.

Their personalities changed. Something fundamental had shifted. Being leaner, fitter and stronger altered the way they felt about themselves. It changed the way they dealt with the world. It sharpened the skills, mental and physical, that they brought to bear in their new daily lives.

Again and again, menopausal women talk of the strange new physical vulnerability they feel at the onset of 'the change', and how that affects them mentally. Building up muscle and stamina can quite literally put iron back in your soul.

STRESS BUSTING

Exercise burns off stress. We take toxins into our body through what we eat and through our polluted environment. But we also produce toxins ourselves. We all know about the 'fight and flight' syndrome. We may not be running away from woolly mammoths any more. But a sharp exchange with a belligerent boss can flood our bodies with exactly the same chemicals that motivated our primeval ancestors. Only we don't work it off by running away from the monster. Instead we sit and stew. And we gradually poison ourselves. Unwanted hormones and excess toxins build up. Tension and stress increase.

WORK IT OUT

Work up a bit of a sweat and you burn off the toxic waste. The way you see your body is going to affect the way you see yourself. Your whole self. And that affects the way you interact with the world. It's not just physical. It's mental.

And it can be made to be positive.

And what's more, that positivity can practically be weighed, measured and bottled. Julius Axelrod, the Nobel prizewinner, came across the 'happy hormone' by accident. He discovered the brain messenger or neurotransmitter, noradrenalin. Noradrenalin alters mood. Calms the mind. Puts a rosy hue on life. People with generally happy personalities have more of it in their bodies than people who are depressed.

The magic of noradrenalin is you can make it for yourself. You don't have to be born with extra-large reserves of it. You don't have to go out and buy it. You don't have to beg, borrow or steal it. Your body produces it naturally. And it does this when you exercise.

Among all human beings, it's the very top athletes who've been measured to produce the most.

Exercise reduces the risk of heart attack. It gives us drive. It increases our vigour. It keeps bones strong and it helps weight control. It'll keep you calmer, more relaxed and so help reduce stress. Regular, moderate exercise adds two years to your life. That's two good years – with improved quality of life in between.

IT'S NEVER TOO LATE TO START

Funnily enough, it's the people who don't exercise at all who have the most to gain in the short term. Just fifteen minutes' brisk walking a day helps enormously. It's not the intensity that counts. It's the regularity.

'Smile,' says cardiologist Dr Jim Rippe, who's director of the Exercise Physiology and Nutrition Laboratory at the University of Massachusetts Medical School. He's not joking. Just the simple muscle spasms that cross your face when you smile automatically get those little neurotransmitters zapping the body and bathing it in their own special elixir.

'Think positive' is another maxim he believes in. Quite literally. When you're ploughing up and down those lanes at your local pool, imagine you're swimming with the dolphins and having a ball. Or if you're on a running machine, fantasise that you're taking magically elongated strides across the tops of the glorious mountains of Nepal.

Play music when you move those muscles. Meditate on your own personal mantra. Make up your own specially tailored phrases and maxims to repeat to yourself as you go along. Focus on a colour you find particularly beautiful. Anything to help lift you out of the everyday. Give yourself your own personalised mini-break from reality.

If you were given an exercise bike for Christmas, put it full square in front of the telly when you're using it. The time will go much quicker.

DOCTOR KNOWS BEST

If you feel it's still all too much, and you're just not sure where to begin, take heart from the GP who started a very unusual treatment programme in his area. He had a number of patients who kept turning up again and again to his surgery whom he just couldn't 'cure'. And they weren't malingerers. They had genuine and serious complaints – depression, under-active thyroids, heavy drinking, heavy smoking, hypertension, cancers, asthmas, obesity, arthritis and diseased lungs.

His prescription was to send them over the road to the fitness centre. And one of his proudest 'cures' was the menopausal woman who'd been on anti-depressants for a long time, but still couldn't stop weeping. After a gentle progression of exercises over a few months, she was able to give her son a run for his money on the rowing machine, covering two and a half thousand metres in ten minutes. She's not weeping any more. And she's off the pills.

STEPPING OUT

Brisk walking is one of the most underrated exercises. It's so simple. It's so cheap. And it's so easy. And though I run a mile from anything which increases worry about body image, walking is great for those of us with the good old pear-shaped rear end. It'll make you fitter and more relaxed. Muscles will tone and tighten. But it's the buttocks, thighs and legs that really benefit. And for some women who might see the beginnings of **stress incontinence** brought on by menopause, the gentle consistent motion around the pelvic region will tone and shape the pelvic floor muscles, and therefore the urethra.

At the University of Oklahoma, a group of women lost a total of four inches from their waists, hips and thighs in just two months after increasing their walking from only two fifteen-minute sessions a week to a total of two hours spread across the seven days. They still ate the same things, but walking radically changed their body contours, *before* they even began to lose weight. **Toning** doesn't mean weight loss. The first is much more important than the second. Get the toning right, and all else will follow in its own good time.

The British Heart Foundation is keen to get us walking. After a brisk walk the **heart rate** becomes slower when you're at rest, so the heart muscle then uses up less oxygen. This means it can pump more efficiently. There's an improvement in the **cholesterol** profile and it can reduce **hypertension**. **Blood circulation** improves and the **immune system** starts working better so you can fight off infections. Plus being in the open exposes you to ultraviolet light that produces Vitamin D within the skin and that helps calcium absorption, a guard against **osteoporosis**.

But more critically for menopausal women, they've found that **bone density** in the lower spine and legs increases too. And one woman I spoke to said it cured her **bloating**. Her legs, hands and joints used to swell right up, but after she set up a daily routine of walking, she's no longer troubled.

'And,' she added, 'I can do it on my own if I feel solitary. Or get together a merry band of us. It's always lovely out in the fresh air. I've even thought of organising a local charity walkathon.'

EXERCISE, FOOD AND FATIGUE

Sedentary animals eat less than moderately active animals and slowly put on weight. Very active animals eat masses and remain svelte. So it is with people too. Cutting back calories alone has been found to help only 5 per cent to 20 per cent of people lose those pounds.

Exercise is essential. You'll digest the food you do eat more thoroughly, so exercise increases your ability to nourish yourself better. You'll sleep better. And perhaps begin to wean yourself off too much tea, coffee, alcohol, refined carbohydrates and sugar. All of which are often used by people who don't exercise, to give themselves those bursts of 'energy' to get through the day. Ironically, those bursts have a high cost. They apparently work in the short term, but deplete energy levels overall. Fatigue sets in again, only worse, so then it's time for another burst of sugar, coffee, chocolate, alcohol – whatever. The vicious circle continues.

Chronic fatigue doesn't have to be our lot. Nor high blood pressure, nor poor intellectual performance. These have all been credited as 'symptoms' of the menopause. They will respond to 'treatment'.

Menopausal women sometimes sense their bodies are becoming alien. But if you change the shape of your body, you change the shape of your life.

CHAPTER 23

Food, glorious food

The Hunzas, the Abkhazians and the Vilcambas live healthily for a very long time. And exercise plays a crucial role in keeping them so fit. We can't mirror that agrarian, subsistence lifestyle and may not want to. But we can certainly help ourselves to keep ticking over physically at a pace which suits us, and stretches us enough to keep our bodies purring in top gear for as long as we need.

Enjoying food is one of life's great joys. But some women put on weight around the menopause and suddenly what used to be a source of great pleasure turns into a minefield.

Our bodies feel out of control. They're subject to all sorts of erratic and apparently uncontrollable sensations. A number of other sensuous delights seem to be shutting down. And on top of all that – food too has to be denied! It's too much.

But it doesn't have to be like that.

First, the weight problem may not be directly related to the menopause. Many of us simply slow down in mid-life. Quite literally. We start, unconsciously, to take things easier. We don't move our bodies quite so energetically. We've worked hard all our lives, so we'll just have that extra helping of lemon meringue pie. We've earned it.

Bouncing around in sweaty aerobics classes is all very well for the youngsters, but for us, something a little more decorous is called for. Like a gentle stroll to the pub.

I'm exaggerating. But you get my drift.

The truth of the matter is that we can never give up. Never give up exercising. Never give up eating carefully. Never give up living to the max.

DITCH THAT DIET

About the only thing we can give up at this time is dieting.
That's one positively healthy move in the right direction. It's
hard to understand why we spend nigh on a hundred million
pounds on the diet industry in this country each year, when
dieting makes you fat. But there you go. There's nowt so
queer as folk.

Our metabolisms do slow down as we grow older so, if
anything, physical activity should increase. And we need to
take extra care about what we put into the furnace to fuel that
activity. Healthy eating is about discipline, not deprivation.

We need to be careful about the 'ordinary' weight that we
pile on at this time, often without realising it, and before it's
too late.

SALTY TALES

But, second, there's the bloating issue. **Water retention** is a
big problem for women whose hormones are swinging like a
pendulum. Your doctor may prescribe you diuretics. You may
prefer to try and cope the natural way. Not least because
artificial diuretics strip the body of potassium (one form of
salt) but leave sodium (another form of salt) – increasing the
imbalance even further.

Water retention is often caused because there's too much
salt in the body. Good old table salt is the villain of the piece.
Basically, we don't need any table salt at all. If you can't give
it up, move over to natural sea salt which you'll get at your
local health store.

There's enough natural sodium in milk, eggs, some vegetables and meat to more than cater for what the body needs.
With a mix of the above in a balanced diet, you'll get two to
three grammes of sodium a day. And that's enough.

But there's nothing like excess. And the Western diet is
nothing if not excessive. Manufacturers shovel salt into

commercially processed convenience foods like bread, butter, cheese, margarine and the thousands of little snacky titbits that help us stagger from one denatured morsel to the next.

The only convenient thing about those foods is that, because their effect on our bodies can be so drastic, there's no confusion about symptoms and treatments. You can't argue with a heart attack or hypertension. Both conditions not helped by our excessive doses of unnecessary salt.

In northern Japan there's a community which lives by the sea and eats an inordinately large amount of salt in their diet, about twenty-five grammes a day. They have one of the worst rates of high blood pressure in the world, and the number one killer in their area is stroke. Inland Japanese who eat much less salt fare much better.

FLOAT AWAY THAT BLOAT

One way to treat bloating is to eat foods that are **natural diuretics**. And to drink them.

When I say drink the foods, I mean juice them. Treat yourself to a juicer. Ask for one for your birthday. Or for Christmas. It's an essential in the kitchen, not a luxury. Juicing is a brilliant way to get all those wonderful nutrients and vitamins and enzymes straight into the system. It seems a contradiction to treat bloating with more liquid, but the quicker and more 'pure' the delivery, the faster the cure.

Watermelons are a natural diuretic. They take away excess fluid from areas prone to cellulite. And they also have a complicated chemical called cucurocitrin, which helps to bring down blood pressure.

Cucumbers and **celery** are other good diuretics. (They also have calcium, by the way, and we know what that's good for.) **Parsley** (yes, you can juice it), **grapes**, fresh **pineapple**, **canteloupe** and **asparagus** have all been mentioned by women with the menopause who've decided to treat their bloating themselves.

SWEET DREAMS

It may come as a surprise to think of your homely, familiar kitchen as a laboratory. But when you start getting into the chemistry of food, you begin to realise that's really not far from the truth.

Take **bananas**. Yes, they're a common or garden fruit that we're so accustomed to, we hardly think of them as out of the ordinary. But they're full of tryptophan. Tryptophan is a **sleep-inducing** amino acid that can have **anti-depressant** qualities. **Milk** and **cheese** also contain tryptophan.

So if your menopause is giving you disturbed sleep and you're feeling unusually blue, eat a banana on an empty stomach just before you go to bed, with a little fruit juice to help digestion.

Some futuristic scientists say, forget drugs; the time will come when we will be playing around with food alone to zap ourselves into altered states of consciousness.

PLAY ON

Pomegranates for instance are known as the food of love. But if you look at just a few of their qualities, you realise they're jam-packed with goodies to make you feel both elated and tranquil at the same time. That kind of cloud-nine feeling.

They contain an alkaloid similar in make-up to the drug mescalin, while at the same time containing substances that have definite calming effects.

This wonderful fruit is also a source of plant hormones which mirror some female hormones. These oestrogen-like substances are in the seeds, so chew them for a while.

Rhubarb also mimics another of our sex hormones, progesterone.

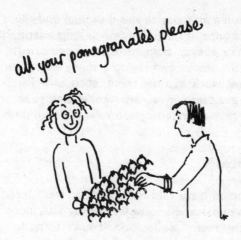

all your pomegranates please

BEAT THE BLUES

Mangoes are good **anti-depressants**. The sheer pleasure of eating a mango is mood-altering enough. But while you're getting carried away on the texture and taste, these 'fruits of heavenly joy' as they're known in Hindu myth are pumping anacardic acid and anacardiol into your system – both of which are closely linked to anti-depressant drugs.

Carrots can be an **aphrodisiac**.

Extracts from **lettuce**, particularly wild lettuce, were used as a truth drug on prisoners of war under interrogation. So powerful is it that in the dim distant past, before we lost all this knowledge, witches, or as we'd call them today, doctors, used to give it to women in childbirth to change their perception of time and pain.

Horseradish is a **stimulant**, as is **fennel**, though that's more mild. **Rosemary** is a stimulant. **Parsley, lettuce** and **cabbage** are **sedatives**.

FOODS FOR MOODS

If you are suffering massive mood swings and other uncomfortable symptoms, it may be worth taking a long, hard look at what you're eating. Some of these foods are going to be subtle in their effects. But if you remove other things from your diet that work against them, such as artificial stimulants, then gradually you can reconstruct your very own internal ecosphere, customised to your individual needs.

BRAIN STRAIN

So many women have told me how they were terrified that their brains had turned to putty during the menopause. 'I can't spell any more,' wailed one. 'I have to write lists, and lists, and more lists. And then I forget where I've put them,' moans another.

Rosemary clears the mind and improves the memory. You can have it applied in oils in aromatherapy sessions, more of which later. But that's expensive. So you could buy a plant at your local garden centre and nurture it, and use it liberally in your cooking. You could also learn how to dry herbs to best protect their essential oils so you have a supply for winter. More time-consuming in the short run than taking a pill, but for those who want to go the natural route, a surer way of knowing exactly what it is you're putting in your body.

COOK ECLECTIC

Food can work for you, rather than against. For instance, you'll want something to perk you up in the middle of the day. So avoid the sedative foods like **lettuce**, **cabbage** and **parsley**.

But they would make a great salad to have at night, particularly if one of your symptoms is **disturbed sleep**.

Though if you're worried about your weight, avoid them altogether. Because they really do sedate. They sedate your thyroid gland, which is the last thing you want if you're trying to kick-start a sluggish metabolism.

For a lunch with zap, stick to stimulating **celery** salad with **fennel** and **rosemary**, plus **grains** or **pulses**. The afternoon will zip by.

YOU CAN'T BEAT THE BEET

The simple old **beetroot** has some pretty amazing benefits. It's claimed to have **anti-ageing** properties, probably because it works on the liver, so tones the whole body. A side-effect is that it helps with **slimming**.

If the liver is overwhelmed with toxins and waste products from a poor diet, it's so busy channelling those out of the system that it doesn't have time to do one of its other main jobs properly. That is, break down fat so it can be properly used, then eliminated. The fat continues to lurk in all those nooks and crannies where we'd rather it didn't, and we lose energy. The alkaloid betaine found in beetroot gets the liver going, cleanses it and increases its ability to fight that fat.

PILL POPPING

One way to boost your diet is to take **vitamins** and **minerals**. They're useful if you're depleted. Though given the range needed, you might feel you've turned into a fully-fledged pill popper.

You might want to supplement your diet that way, or alternatively concentrate on eating foods rich in the particular vitamins or minerals you've decided you need.

It is possible to get everything from a healthy diet. Some nutritionists are taking the radical view that if, alongside other changes like diet and exercise, the menopausal woman eats enough of the foods that closely mimic oestrogen compounds, that could be a viable alternative to taking HRT.

EAT FOR HEALTH

So many of the problems of menopause are caused simply by sudden **food intolerances** and **sugar imbalances**. Both can be dealt with by healthy eating.

'Optimum nutrition' is the latest buzz in the world of food experts. Being fully 'nutrified' is when your body is working to its top capacity – because it has all the ingredients it needs to achieve peak performance. And that is not about running a mile in four minutes. It's about putting the right ingredients into the system in order to maximise your own personal potential – whatever that might be. It's something that's a lot more rare than many of us realise.

Take the following menu. It's an average wholefood diet for a day, and it'll give you everything you need:

Get up and go
A balanced set of meals could include a breakfast of a delicious and crunchy mixture of wholegrain cereals (good quality muesli) with bananas and soya milk.

Snack attack
Snack on raw vegetables, nuts, seeds and fruit and wholemeal rolls, to bridge that gap.

Eat energy
Toss some salmon salad with watercress, baby leeks, red peppers and pumpkin seeds for lunch.

Saving staples
And for supper have shepherd's pie made from lentils, with

creamed potatoes, sprinkled with cheese and cooked till lightly golden brown.

Treat time
End up with a symphony of hazelnut and apricot yoghurt, using natural live yoghurt.

It's balanced. It's healthy and it's free of many of the foodstuffs that work against you rather than for you.

SLOWLY DOES IT

Getting rid of poor food in the diet takes time. It's taken us a lifetime to get used to it. It takes a while to wean ourselves off it. But it's worth it. If you think your diet's lacking and want to start forging a bedrock of solid nutrition to draw on, allow for at least a year to get up to full potential.

It's hard, if not well nigh impossible, to give up pleasures like **alcohol**, **tea**, **coffee**, **cola** drinks and **chocolate**. But they are all artificial stimulants and put enormous strain on the adrenal glands.

Drinking **alcohol** with the wild abandon we had in our youth begins to pall, not least when our bodies don't seem to have the same ability to take it. There's just that one morning too many when the bounce-back fails to materialise. The days of wine and roses needn't be entirely over. But more roses and less wine would help.

TREASURE TROVE

During the menopause the body becomes increasingly dependent on the small, but significant, amounts of oestrogen that the adrenals can produce. The ovaries have virtually packed up, so they can be relied on less and less.

Stress your adrenals and you're wasting a precious resource.

In fact, if you're a coffee-drinking smoker who takes no exercise and also drinks alcohol, going the 'optimum nutrition' route is not for you. Your body just wouldn't have a chance to build resources. Some damage already inflicted becomes irreversible. Though it's never too late to change that which isn't.

As we age, the adrenals begin to lose their rapid response. They still go on working, otherwise we'd collapse entirely. But they just don't have quite the same power they've had before. So at the very time when we need them in tiptop condition, by continuing to take in artificial stimulants we're sabotaging the very thing we need most.

Taking the stimulants out of your diet helps clear the head. You can think more clearly. Coping with daily stress levels becomes easier.

YOU CAN MAKE IT

Wholewheat bread, cucumber, alfalfa and **citrus fruits** all contain oestrogen-type compounds. Boost your diet with them, and you may boost your ability to manufacture your own oestrogen.

It's said that **Evening Primrose Oil** helps with oestrogen manufacture, along with **Vitamin E.** As do vital oils from fresh **nuts, seeds** and **wholegrains** – **soya, chickpeas** and **lentils** which have essential fatty acids similar to Evening Primrose Oil. They also work on the cardiovascular system, giving you protection similar to that of HRT.

These plants and foods which contain substances similar to the female hormones are made up of phyto-oestrogens. These are compounds that mimic those precious hormones that the menopausal woman is gradually losing. If we put enough of them in our diets, we should significantly affect our ability to go on producing what we need.

THE GOOD GUYS AND THE BAD GUYS

The body makes three types of oestrogen: 'good' oestrogen – 'oestriol'; bad oestrogen – 'oestradiol', and 'oestrone', which converts the 'bad' oestrogen into 'good' oestrogen.

The first 'good' oestrogen, oestriol, is non-carcinogenic. Vegetarian diets have been proved to produce much higher levels of 'good' oestriol than those including meat.

If you want to encourage your body to produce more 'good' oestrogen, then you need lots of **Vitamin B**, because that's what it takes to do it.

And Vitamin B means mood foods. The B Vitamins help the adrenals. They also affect the level of glucose in the body, which has an immediate impact on your emotional state. If you get hit by the blues more than usual during your menopause, check your Vitamin B intake. Stimulants, stress, antibiotics and HRT all hoover up the B Vitamins. You can boost them in your diet by eating more **green vegetables** (raw is great), **nuts**, **seeds**, **brewer's yeast**, **wheat germ** and **wholegrains**.

BOWEL BEAUTIFUL

The B Vitamins are made by the intestinal flora in your bowel. Keep that healthy and your body can go on producing what you need. Antibiotics wipe out the delicate lining, and are one of the reasons you might find taking them slightly depressing. So supplement with B Vitamins if you have to take a course. **Live yoghurt** keeps the flora healthy, so eat that. But whether you buy it from a wholefood store or from a supermarket, make sure the label says it really is 'live', because most yoghurts are very dead.

THE BARE BONES OF IT

We are all children of our times. And what's now coming home to roost with a vengeance is the fall-out from the Twiggy phenomenon. There's a whole generation of women who have lived their adult lives crashing from one diet to the next. These women may not be thin. With all their efforts they may never have been thin. But they are almost certainly malnourished. **Diets** don't work. Healthy eating does.

Some nutritionists predict that many of these women will be among the osteoporosis sufferers of the future. For decades they've denied their bodies the nutrients essential to metabolise the vitamins and minerals that build healthy tissue, strong bones, and a durable organism.

Imagine the woman on a depleted diet, 'shooting up' with coffee and cigarettes to stop eating. Torturing herself with small portions of probably the wrong foods. Or grinding through meal after meal of poor quality mass-produced diet drinks or biscuit substitutes. Inevitably there are mood swings; inevitably there are binges of foods rich in sugars to get through the lows, including sweets, chocolate and alcohol. And those stimulants, in their turn, immediately create more lows. It wreaks a kind of damage that can take years to show.

BONE-LOADING

You can literally load your bones with **calcium**. The single most sure way is by doing 'bone-loading' exercises. That's the latest jargon for what we've always called weight-bearing exercise. Brisk walking. Jogging. Running. Anything that makes the skeleton work. Good exercise is one of the greatest protections you can ever have against osteoporosis, as it helps the body absorb the calcium in your food.

But you have to get the calcium into the body in the first place. Foods high in calcium are **parsley, spinach, water-**

cress, **chickpeas**, **haricot beans**, **kidney beans**, **dried figs**, **broccoli**, **tofu** (bean curd), **whole lemons**, **almonds**, **brazil nuts**, **sesame seeds**, **peanuts** and **muesli**. Once there, **Vitamin D** helps its absorption.

Try a raw broccoli and raw spinach salad, sprinkled with almonds and sesame seed oil.

Or a bean salad with watercress, brazil nuts and lemon-flavoured dressing containing slivers of tangy zest from the lemon skin with a little honey.

Loadsacalcium.

Oestrogen protects your calcium. You need oestrogen for a number of things, and one of those is to guard your calcium to make sure it reaches the parts of the body where it'll do most good. You can eat all the calcium you need, but if you don't have enough oestrogen to get it into your bone tissue, you can lose it through your urine. Or even worse, it may end up on your artery walls, or in your joints, contributing to arthritis.

Another thing that oestrogen does in relation to the bones is to stop the production of too much parathyroid. Parathyroid's OK in small doses, but it's a hormone that strips calcium from the bone and deposits it in the blood. Good for the blood – poor for the skeleton.

When there's less oestrogen, there's more parathyroid. So the menopausal woman has to be extra vigilant. The damage caused as it leaches calcium from the living bone tissue is made worse by excessive use of stimulants.

Magnesium plays an important part in calcium uptake. You need the two working in tandem.

People think that dairy foods are good for you because they're rich in calcium. But they have virtually no magnesium at all, plus they're often too rich in fats, and plus they're mucous-producing. Better to return to the nuts and seeds and green leafy vegetables which have a good balance of both. Herbs containing both are **nettle**, **comfrey**, **oatstraw**, and **horsetail**. Magnesium and calcium also work together to increase the alkaline quality of the blood which helps improve the function of all cells.

Keep **protein** levels low. Too much protein creates a heavily acid blood. Even more calcium is taken from the bones in order to offset that acid.

SUPER ALGAE

As we've heard, Linda, the woman who underwent surgery after a long and painful menopause, said she's trying out Super Blue-Green Algae to balance out her menopausal symptoms. Whether by chance or design, she's lit on a food which has been measured as having the highest quality nutrient density of almost anything else on the planet, including meat. She's come across a compound that is higher in protein than almost any other food, but so natural and easily digestible that it doesn't cause damage at the same time.

Super Blue-Green Algae are packed with Vitamin B complex. Vitamin B12, is one of the vitamins that are particularly helpful where 'women's problems' are concerned. It is also the only vitamin that the body cannot manufacture itself, so it does have to be taken in through diet. The algae also contain Vitamin A, iron and a goodly range of minerals and trace elements.

They're a bit like spinach, and are a concentrated way of eating greens. They can be sprinkled on salads and vegetables or soup, and also taken in capsule form.

They've been a staple food for many ancient civilisations. The Mayans and Aztecs harvested and dried them. Even today the Mexicans make biscuits of them for their children. And in India, in a new health initiative, they're being put into noodles for children.

They've got a particularly high profile among athletes who apparently take them in large doses because help their stamina. Some scientists are so excited about them that they say one day they're going to feed the world.

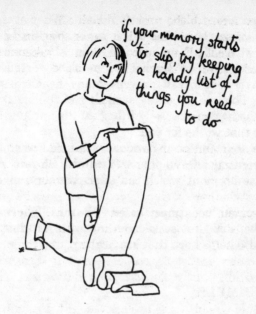

if your memory starts to slip, try keeping a handy list of things you need to do

LOAD UP, LOAD UP

The Japanese have a diet high in foods which promote the production of oestrogen, and it's been found that Japanese village women get few **hot flushes**. In the UK, up to three-quarters of menopausal women have them, especially those who're thin. You might find that **Vitamin E** combined with **Vitamin C** helps.

Many doctors deny that **aching joints** are a menopausal symptom, though there are a number of women who could put them right. The reason for the pain could be the development of food intolerances, due to the upheavals in the rest of the body.

Wheat and **dairy foods** are often the culprits. If you switch to **rye**, **oats**, **barley**, **brown rice** and **soya** products, the pain could lessen. Two other things that help are **Evening Primrose Oil** and **fish oils**.

Oestrogen keeps blood vessels dilated. When it declines, your blood vessels thin. And this is never so critical as in the skull area where it can produce the **headaches** some women have. **Vitamin B3**, or niacin, widens blood vessels and, if taken early enough, can prevent many headaches before they start. Though, of course, widening of the blood vessels can at the same time cause hot flushes. Play around till you find a dose that works for you.

Memory loss and **poor concentration** can be among the most disorienting of symptoms. **Vitamin B5** and **choline** work on the hormone which can affect memory, giving it a boost.

Some women use unperfumed **Vitamin E cream** for **vaginal dryness**, but supplementing with **Vitamins A, C** and **zinc** also helps keep the skin healthy.

KEEP IT SIMPLE

It's easy to be blinded by science with all the food facts now circulating. It takes time to assimilate them into your life, let alone your body.

It can be overwhelming, even confusing, with all the different vitamins and minerals. But these days there are excellent products in healthfood stores which can give you a combination of the lot in one high-nutrient drink or food supplement. To begin with, and before you start your own experiments, it can make the whole thing so much simpler.

There are more and more nutritionists around who have a grasp of the fine tuning necessary for the menopause. Because in fact different vitamins may be necessary at different stages of the menopause. And, indeed, some which should be taken at the beginning, shouldn't be taken towards the end, and vice versa.

There are two good organisations that can help. One is the Women's Nutritional Advisory Service, who will only ever prescribe a course of nutritional supplements that have been scientifically tested. They have a postal and telephone service.

And there's also the Institute of Optimum Nutrition, an independent charity. This is a pioneering organisation at the very forefront of the latest in food and nutrition. They have a training programme and therefore a network of fully qualified nutritionists all over the country, who work as consultants.

BACK TO THE FUTURE

Our bodies are programmed to keep us alive from one moment to the next. If a body 'thinks' at all, it doesn't 'think' beyond the next second. Is there enough oxygen to feed the brain? Is there enough life force to propel the metabolism? It will do only that which is essential for life in the present.

A poor diet takes time to deplete us. Bad lifestyles have a cumulative effect over the years. Our bodies, though, have no concern for that. They don't 'think' ten, twenty, thirty years down the road.

But we can.

CHAPTER 24

The do-it-yourself
keep-fit kit

Looking good. Feeling fit. Bounding with energy. That's how
to live life. And we can most of the time. Especially when
we're on top of things and feeling 'up'. There are times,
though, during the menopause when that can prove an
elusive state of body and mind. But lay the ground right, and
it's possible to maintain peak condition right through 'the
change'.

The food you eat and the exercise you take are two of the
most important ingredients. Vitality is there for the taking.
Get those right, and many of the symptoms that cause
irritability and tiredness will ease.

But as well as exercise and healthy eating, there are the
many therapies, treatments and remedies available from the
world of complementary medicine.

One woman who treats her menopausal patients with
acupressure said, 'What happens is they suddenly want to
start taking care of themselves. They can't understand why
they feel so awful. Why they suddenly lack confidence and
have no energy. Just coming here and talking about it helps
enormously. Often for the first time someone else is listening,
and understands. And they're getting nurtured and cared for
in a way they haven't before. Just the human contact is
therapeutic, let alone the acupressure.'

The smorgasbord of therapies collected in this chapter is
just a taster. There are many more.

All of them can offer something specifically for menopausal
women, many of whom don't go to the doctor. That doesn't

mean they don't have symptoms. Perhaps their symptoms are just not that disruptive. They may want to self-treat instead. These therapies are to be dipped into and experimented with. You might find just the thing to relieve that one little niggle that has come on since your menopause started.

Many remedies that I mention are now so well known that they've become mainstream. Some of them are more unusual. But what seems a little weird today could become conventional tomorrow.

Many GPs include complementary medicine in their NHS practices. These therapies are exactly what the name implies, complementary, and will work in tandem with treatment you are getting from your doctor.

Some techniques are based on ancient knowledge, going back thousands of years. All of them offer a great reservoir of information and healing.

The range of choice can leave you a bit nonplussed to begin with. The thing to do is consider them all with an open mind. Some will appear wacky, or just not for you, while others might ring a bell. The ones worth considering are the ones you think you'd be most comfortable giving a try. Those you gravitate to naturally are the ones that you will be most in sympathy with, and they are the ones that will probably do the greatest good.

GO FOR THE STRETCH – YOGA

My neighbour does a quick blast of yoga three times a day before each meal. She says it keeps her appetite perky. She's ninety-two.

Yoga isn't about tying yourself in knots, and turning yourself inside out. It's about gentle stretching and deep breathing.

It was developed over four thousand years ago in India and it works on both the body and the mind. Basically its aim is to still the mind, but in order to do that, you first have to still the body. So you work on the body, but the by-product is a calming, relaxing feeling that leaves you better equipped for the daily round.

Yoga aims for physical and mental control by slowly and gently putting the body through a series of postures or asanas. These are basic body positions that you curl, and curve, and stretch into – and then hold still. The emphasis is on going at your own pace, doing what you can do and aiming for no more. Gradually, each curl and curve and stretch will extend a little more till your muscles and joints become more flexible and there is a greater fluidity to all your movements, both in the class and out.

What's important is not to be disheartened when you see the eighty-year-old lady next to you doing the splits. She's probably been gradually stretching her hip, thigh and groin muscles for twenty years. It takes time. And where you're at is good enough for now. You're on the right track.

When dealing with the menopause, yoga teachers would encourage you to do daily practice. Five minutes a day is better than two hours once a week.

The menopause is a natural state brought about by fluctuations in hormones produced by the endocrine system. You can help that endocrine system perform more smoothly by doing postures that increase the flow of blood around the **neck**, where important glands are located. These postures are called inversions, and for the expert yoga student can include **shoulder stands**. For the novice, you start simply by lying on the floor and lifting your legs up against a wall, or even sofa. It can be that simple.

Active postures are encouraged for complaints like **depression** and **stress**, so for those you'd do basic **standing postures** and **stretches**.

Most important is the relaxation period at the end of the class, when for about four or five minutes you do *nothing*. Giving yourself permission to do absolutely nothing can take a while. It's not something we're used to.

In India there are yogis who can do incredible contortions and movements, but they have been working on their bodies from babyhood. Yogis can achieve profoundly deep meditative states, so deep that they can actually slow down all their internal body processes to what seems an alarming degree.

They retreat to caves and can stay for extraordinarily long periods in the cool, dark interiors in a sort of suspended animation. The cool and the dark of the cave offers a form of sensory deprivation which cuts out stimuli from the surroundings. That means their bodies are under minimum stress, with no demands internally or externally.

Some have been known to stay in this state for months. Without food or water. In fact, it's a delicate balance because they do have to keep their life force at the most minimal level in order not to allow their vital signs to slow to such a degree that they appear dead. Because then the worms begin to eat them.

The menopause can be bad. But let's hope it's not so bad that you'd want to crawl into a black hole. Certainly yoga, with its focus on breathing and relaxation, can be immensely steadying.

Yoga is so widespread now that you can probably pick up a class at your local leisure centre. If they don't have them, ask for one. You'd be surprised at the demand.

Useful addresses
Yoga for Health Foundation, Ickwell Bury, Ickwell Green, Nr Biggleswade, Beds SG18 9ES. Tel: 0767 627271.

Iyengar Yoga Institute, 223a Randolph Avenue, London W9 1NL. Tel: 071 624 3080.

LESS IS MORE – HOMEOPATHY: THE MAGIC OF THE INFINITESIMAL

'I use sepia for the sag,' said the homeopath describing his specific remedies for the menopause.

Charming. But effective. Sepia treats a complete depletion

of energy. Those moments when everything overwhelms and it all feels too much.

Many women who can't take HRT for medical reasons, because of risk of high blood pressure or thrombosis, turn to this gentle form of medication.

Homeopathy is one of the most subtle of all complementary medicines. It's important to remember that practitioners focus on the individual as a whole. So even if you go to a homeopath with 'sag' symptoms, you might be given a different remedy than sepia, simply because there's no one cure for each and every individual.

And you'll be asked a long list of questions, like whether you prefer spicy or bland foods, whether you like to be indoors or out. Or what time you wake up in the night. This way your unique and individual profile is built up and the homeopath gets a comprehensive understanding of the way your body ticks.

Homeopathy works on a principle discovered at the turn of the eighteenth century. The idea is that the more minute the dose of medicine given to you, the more powerful its effect will be. Remedies are diluted and diluted, sometimes till there is only a fraction of the original substance left – potencies can be reduced to one part in ten million. It's an idea that turns conventional medicine on its head. But they both work in their own ways. It's for you to choose which route you want to try.

Homeopathy has discovered that substances which are poisonous in their natural state can be used to cure. But they will cure only those ailments that they themselves cause. 'Let like be treated by like' is one of homeopathy's maxims. A homeopath will prescribe a substance which, if taken in massive doses, produces the very symptoms you're trying to get rid of.

Symptoms are important signposts. They show that the body's own natural defences are tackling the underlying illness. But they are just the physical manifestation of the real problem.

By using a homeopathic remedy, from a plant, animal or mineral extract which brings on the same symptoms as the disease, the natural defences in the body are triggered so that the body's own healing power combats whatever your illness might be. But homeopathy uses infinitesimally small quantities, so there are no major side-effects.

A good remedy for **hot flushes** is **Lachesis**. And **Pulsatilla** helps with tearful, **weepy spells**. But again all the treatments are so carefully designed for the individual that you might find yourself coming away with something altogether different.

Homeopathy is one of the few complementary medicines where you may have problems finding someone who will treat you if you are already on HRT. I've spoken to some homeopaths who will treat, because they feel something is better than nothing. But even they are reluctant. Most won't. The HRT acts as an antidote, blocking the effect of the homeopathic remedy. Its ability to work freely on the system is compromised and so even if there is a result, it'll be limited.

If you're interested, ask your GP, because homeopathy is available in some areas on the NHS. More and more people are trying it. Sales of homeopathic products doubled from £6 million in the mid Eighties to £15 million by the beginning of the Nineties.

Useful addresses
The Society of Homeopaths, 2 Artizan Road, Northampton NN1 4HU. Tel: 0604 21400. Fax: 0604 22622.

STAND TALL AND TAKE THE WORLD IN YOUR STRIDE – THE ALEXANDER TECHNIQUE

Watch young children at rest and at play. So many of them move with grace. There is an alertness and poise that allows them to sit, stand and run with a dynamic fluidity that seems long gone from our older bodies.

Where does it go? How do we lose it? Through bad habits collected over the years is how. The slouch, the droop, the couch potato.

The Alexander Technique quite literally takes us back to childhood and teaches us to find again the best way to inhabit our skins. It focuses on the spine initially and then the whole skeleton, encouraging people to shake out ingrained patterns of standing and sitting that twist and warp. You will rediscover the posture that most truly reflects you at your most vital and alive.

Most of us have developed physical short cuts to what we think of as relaxation. But they aren't. They're just ingrained physical responses which interfere with our natural coordination and functioning. We become disconnected. We find ourselves reacting automatically, harming and even reducing our energy and effectiveness.

The Alexander Technique is basically a way of rediscovering that plumb-line that runs from the very tip of our heads to the base of our spines. That pure line between you and gravity. The way our bodies twist and contort around that line is a measure of our very dysfunction. Find that line, straighten out your body, and it's surprising how it can straighten out other things in your life.

The integration of our system as a whole is primarily affected by our head, neck and back coordination. Get that wrong and you get **headaches**, **backaches**, **stiff necks** and **shoulders**. These are general lurgies that can undermine our sense of well-being, though they're often not so bad that we can quite put our finger on exactly what it is that is causing the problem. Or really get around to doing something constructive about it.

But they can cause more than just irritating aches and pains. They can have a very real effect on poise, our sense of being in touch with our bodies, and our levels of vitality. Body and mind weave together inextricably. Lack of physical poise can affect our state of mind and our ability to cope.

The therapy is deceptively simple. The therapist will just

gently handle your head and neck, and then your whole body, your shoulders, chest, pelvis, legs and feet, to correct imbalances.

The Alexander Technique is particularly good for the menopausal woman who feels quite literally weighed down with symptoms. Stand tall, and you'll feel tall. Stand straight and you can look the world in the eye again.

Useful addresses
Society of Teachers of the Alexander Technique, 10 London House, 266 Fulham Road, London SW10 9EL. Tel: 071 351 0828.

SUPERB HERBS

It's comforting to know that modern drug companies spend millions of dollars of their profits every year trying to find ways to mimic and replicate medicinal compounds found growing in the wild. It's a reassuring vote of confidence in nature.

The first doctors were all herbalists. And they knew their stuff. One of the earliest books in the West documenting herbal remedies was written in Greece in 400BC. But it wasn't until the first century AD that Dioscorides put together a definitive list of over six hundred plants, all to be used for medical purposes.

There are many herbs that act as **uterine tonics**. Some have oestrogen-like effects, and some work like progesterone, so they can be taken in combination to mimic and support our own natural menstrual cycle.

Two of the most exciting are those which can be taken as tinctures. The first is called **Vitex agnus castus**, and the second is **Dong quai**.

Vitex agnus castus comes from the chaste tree plant. It isn't in itself a progesterone, but it encourages the production of progesterone. As a uterine tonic, it helps to clear away the lining of the womb that is part of every normal period.

151

You can take it every day throughout your whole cycle. It's a hormonal stabiliser and normaliser, so it works to ensure that hormones are produced in the right ratios.

Dong quai tincture is a powerful uterine tonic with oestrogen-like properties which encourages the production of your own natural oestrogen. Take this only for the first three weeks of your cycle, not when you start to bleed. If your cycles are becoming irregular, take it for as long as the spell of non-bleeding lasts. Then when you do start a period, stop the Dong quai, and just keep going with Vitex in its usual daily dose.

Anyone on HRT will notice the similarities in the hormonal balancing act.

There are other herbs which mirror our female hormones, and influence the entire pelvic region. Beware; they can taste foul. But they do work.

Black cohosh is one of them and is often used to treat **weakness** and **depression**. It's a root which, like Dong quai, has oestrogen-like properties. As an **anti-spasmodic** and **sedative**, it can help with **cramps** and calm **tensions**, and is good when combined with Vitex.

It could also be combined with another herb, **wild yam**. That contains substances vital to the production of progesterone. **Wild yam** benefits the **uterus** and **soothes the nerves**.

Squaw vine is a big star in American Indian medicine. It's an excellent all-over body tonic, but especially for the uterus. It is used to treat **painful heavy periods** and combines as a diuretic too, so is good for **bloating**. As is **dandelion**, which is one of the best, along with **nettle**.

Use **motherwort** if you're aiming to treat the emotional upsets and anxieties that can surround menopause. It seems to work on **attitude**, but helps with **hot flushes** too.

Something else for **hot flushes** is **sage**. Drink it as a tea. Again, it's got a strong taste so don't let it stew. Make an infusion and have it straight away. It's good for the sweats.

Cramp bark is another herb that is used by American native Indians. It relaxes, and **releases tension**, so is good if you're under pressure and stress. And it is also good for pale and **scanty periods**.

Angelica root is a stimulant and general tonic, often prescribed to restore **confidence** and a sense of **well-being**. **Liquorice root** stimulates **hormone function**. It has compounds similar to oestrogen. And **Pennyroyal** contains substances similar to progesterone.

The above is just a small cross-section of what's available. Herbs usually have to be taken for two weeks or so before their beneficial effects begin to show.

Take care if you're both menopausal and pregnant. Some of these herbs really do evacuate the womb and that may not be what you want. A good herbalist will identify and personalise what's most appropriate for you.

Useful addresses

National Institute of Medical Herbalists, 9 Palace Gate, Exeter EX1 1JA. Tel: 0392 426022.

British Herbal Medicine Association, Field House, Lye Hole Lane, Redhill, Avon BS18 7TB. Tel: 0934 862994.

Neal's Yard Remedies, 15 Neal's Yard, Covent Garden, London WC2H 9DP. Tel: 071 379 7222.

Iden Croft Herbs, Frittenden Road, Staplehurst, Kent TN12 0DH. Tel: 0580 891432.

Baldwin & Co, 173 Walworth Road, London SE17 1RW. Tel: 071 703 5550.

A LIFE ON THE OCEAN BRINE – FLOATING: THE ONLY WAY TO GROW

'Floating', as it's known among aficionados, is one of the best stress busters in the business. It's hard to believe you can go for an ocean dip right in the middle of many of our towns and cities – but it's become a reality.

Floating can seem a little daunting to the uninitiated, but it's worth a try.

A 'float tank' is like a space capsule full of water saturated with about half a ton of Epsom salts. It's like the sea – only more so. The nearest real-life equivalent is the Dead Sea, an enormous natural health spa in its own right.

The salt supports you on the surface of the water, which is only about eight inches deep, so non-swimmers needn't worry. Once you're inside, the door is closed so that you are in the complete dark. You can have taped music, from Vivaldi to Navaho bellchimes to the mating calls of whales. Or you can choose complete silence. You lie in the warm water and float. It's that simple.

Floating creates biochemical changes in the nervous system. Brain biochemistry is simply another piece of jargon for describing the processes that make us tick as human beings. Certain brain chemicals make us shy or competitive, afraid or anxious, happy, sleepy, depressed, irritated and so on. They play a major role in stress. They sexually arouse us, give us vitality, or swamp our system when we fall in love.

You can alter and regulate your own brain chemicals. So you can alter and regulate your own behaviour.

Among many other things, floating lowers the levels of hormones which are linked to stress and stress-related illnesses. Also the 'happy' hormones, endorphins, are released in abundance, which probably explains the rather spaced-out, super-relaxed state you emerge in.

There are many theories about what goes on in the body when it's freed from the weight of gravity – which is what happens in a flotation tank. Whatever it is, you come out so relaxed it's unwise to get straight into a car if you're driving. Give yourself ten to fifteen minutes 'decompression' time.

Thankfully, our bodies are constantly responding to that centrifugal tug generated from the centre of our whirling planet. Without it, we'd be beamed up so fast that Mr Spock wouldn't know what hit him. But gravity can have its drawbacks. A holiday from it now and again gives the body a bit of a breather.

Ninety per cent of what goes on inside our bodies is in sole response to gravity. Take away the gravity, and you free up all that energy which is tied down dealing with the non-stop pull.

The bulk of stimuli absorbed by the nervous system is from muscular activity inevitably forced into constant dialogue with the surrounding force field. All our perceptions and sensations take place against this backdrop. Give the body a break and you give your nervous system a break too.

You are mentally and physically liberated after a float because your mind and body have not had to process the constant stream of information that being locked into gravity requires.

When the body functions under normal gravitational pressure, the cardiovascular system, for instance, is working under strain. Our bodies try to compensate, and inevitably adopt rigid postures, which can result in localised muscular tension. As you float, you find your skeleton, muscles and joints automatically reverting to naturally relaxed and loose poses.

Float fanatics promise that flotation tanks will cure everything under the sun from **high blood pressure** to **ulcers**. That's as may be. What they do, without doubt, is take the body back to a state of such relaxed bliss that whatever your presenting symptom may be, for a brief moment the body seems to experience a state of true healing. Stop the mind. Stop the stress. Stop the pain. Let the body have the last word. It often knows best. And it's often the quickest healer.

Useful addresses
Flotation Tank Association, Tel: 0923 285868.

Aquatonics (also builds tanks), 4 Wellington Close, Ledbury Road, London W11 2AN. Tel: 071 229 1123.

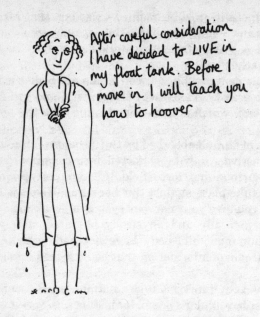

After careful consideration I have decided to LIVE in my float tank. Before I move in I will teach you how to hoover

PUTTING YOUR BEST FOOT FORWARD – REFLEXOLOGY

Reflexology is one of those therapies which has been around for thousands and thousands of years. It's a deep massage system that concentrates on the soles of the feet.

All our nerves travel on pathways around the body. Different nerves service different organs. This network produces a transit system through the body of channels of energy. Sometimes these channels get blocked. All of them pass through the sole of the foot. Find the right spot on the sole of the foot, massage it, and you will release that block, wherever it is in the body.

If you look at a reflexologist's chart of the feet, it is like a map of your body. Different areas of the feet correspond to different areas of the body. The menopausal woman may be diagnosed as having an under-active pituitary gland, so she'll find that the central area of skin on the sole of her big toes will be gently massaged. That's where the nerve endings from the pituitary surface on the feet.

The reflexologist may decide to stimulate the adrenal glands to encourage them to continue oestrogen production after the ovaries have stopped. So the area tucked under the ball of the foot gets the treatment.

Reflexology is particularly good for **bad circulation**, giving a boost to poor blood flow. It stimulates the body's detoxification process, cleansing, renewing and revitalising on a very deep level. It's particularly good as a preventative measure as it stimulates the body's own healing process. And it's best taken in a course of treatment, maybe once a week for six weeks.

Treatments usually last around forty minutes to an hour. The reflexologist may use a basic unperfumed talc dusted on to the feet to give an easy surface to work on, or maybe oils. Reflexology doesn't tickle. It soothes and relaxes.

It's so successful as an anaesthetic that it's offered as pain relief instead of drugs at the Middlesex Hospital in Central London. An enlightened example of complementary and mainstream medicine working together.

It also works as a general **relaxant**, but it's particularly

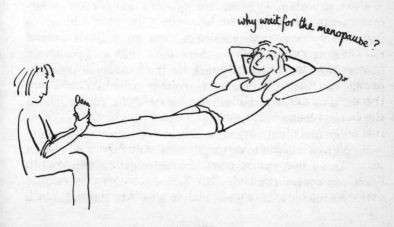

why wait for the menopause?

successful for **bad headaches** and **migraines**, which can be a trial during menopause.

It's also often used in treating **addictions**, not that the menopausal woman is necessarily an addictive personality. But as we know, some women make sweeping changes at menopause – re-assessing and re-organising their life and priorities. Letting go of a marriage, job or relationship can be similar to getting rid of other destructive patterns like smoking, excessive alcohol use or even chocolate addiction.

Reflexology increases a sense of well-being that lessens tension and can make you feel good about yourself.

Useful addresses
The British School of Reflexology, 92 Sheering Road, Old Harlow, Essex CM17 OJW. Tel: 0279 429060.

AROMATHERAPY

It's well known that in spring a young man's fancy is supposed to turn from an abiding interest in the hewing of wood, the tending of sheep and the relative chances of his team in the football league – to sex. This has been put down to a rising of the sap. It's probably true.

When the plant kingdom springs into action after a dormant winter, the aroma can be heady. The gift of a bunch of flowers may carry more messages than we realise – women have oestrogen receptors in their noses that will positively quiver with delight as they pick up the oestrogen-like compounds in the plants. Those compounds travel straight into the nervous system and, all else being equal, can trigger a rise in the libido.

History has kindly drawn a delicate veil over what young women are supposed to do at this time, but there's no reason not to think that they too are looking to get their rocks off. Scent can transport us.

For thousands of years, plants and the essential oils

distilled from them have been used to heal, to soothe, to stimulate, to invoke the gods and cast spells. Essential oils are the life-blood of the plant.

They can be used as beauty treatments. **Skin tone** can be lost at the menopause, and never so much as on the face and neck. Cleopatra, who was a chemist and scholar in her free time, used **cedar wood** and **sandalwood** oils as a face mask to rejuvenate her skin. Both of them also **revitalise the spirits**.

She could also have used a blend of **neroli**, **myrrh**, **rose**, **frankincense** and **lavender**. They help regenerate the **growth of cells**. Massage a blend of them into the skin every night and the glow soon returns. Eight drops of frankincense or myrrh, fourteen drops of lavender and three drops of neroli mixed with fifty millilitres of unscented cosmetic oil will be a real tonic.

Aromatherapy helps even out moods and the **emotions**. Nothing brings back a memory, or an atmosphere, so powerfully as a sudden waft of a scent that takes us back in time.

Our sense of scent seems to work so profoundly on our memory banks that it goes further than just the intellect. It's as if our whole body responds on an almost molecular level. Emotions are buried deep. Aromatherapy seems to have the power to reach into the chaos of the jangled nervous system and, by gentle and subtle means, restore our inner sense of well-being.

Essential oils relax the nervous system, stimulate the **circulation**, lift **depression**, aid in the **detoxification** of the body, and generally ease the lurking aches and pains caused by our busy and hurried lives. Some extracts from plants have been found to be very similar in form to the female hormones. **Clary**, **rose** and **fennel** have all been mentioned before. They work particularly well on 'female problems'.

Essential oils are extracted from different parts of the plant. Some come from resins; others from herbs, flowers and spices.

They're very powerful. You only need a drop or two, mixed in with a good quality, unscented body oil. They travel directly to the brain when inhaled and have deep penetrative powers through the skin when used in massage.

For the menopausal woman buffeted by swings of mood and a body that can at times seem out of control, a gentle massage with oils can help **stress**, **tension**, **fluid retention**, **depression** and **headaches**.

Useful addresses
International Federation of Aromatherapists, Royal Masonic Hospital, Ravenscourt Park, London W6 OTN. Tel: 081 846 8066.

GETTING DOWN TO ESSENTIALS – BURNING THE MIDNIGHT OIL

Aromatics can make you go out of your mind. This can be useful. Massaging oils into the skin is aromatherapy. Burning an oil for its heady scent is aromatics. The two are completely different in their effects.

For instance, oil of **geranium** when used as an aromatherapy massage oil will work as a **diuretic**, so is good for **bloating**, **eczema** and **anxiety**. But *burn* it and it can 'bring on acts of uncharacteristic rashness'.

Next time you have some particularly stuffy friends round for supper, you might want to erect a little shrine to orgiastic pantheism by putting some in an incense burner on the sideboard.

You are entering the realms of the magical when you play around with burning essential oils. The traditional churches knew a trick or two with their smells and bells. We shouldn't lose sight of the fact that these scents were designed to heighten religious experience, and in some cases bring on religious ecstasies.

Tibetan lamas mix fabulously complex variations of herbs

and flowers into an incense which focuses the mind for meditation. In the olden days, temple prostitutes would combine the most potent of scents to come up with an aroma that was an irresistible aphrodisiac.

Pot pourris litter our homes for weeks after Christmas and birthdays. And many of us use pomanders, sachets and room sprays, all of which enhance the scent of the environment and often lift our mood.

But it's possible to personalise aromatics by buying a small number of oils and a burner, and simply experimenting to find what works for you.

Burning **neroli** can set your brain into full-tilt alert. But if you want to wind down, use **white rose** which will induce a delicious sense of lethargy and **repose**.

Moods can disappear. Pessimism turn to optimism. You can turn *up* your level of consciousness, or turn it *down*. For the menopausal woman confused by mood swings a knowledge of aromatics, or how to manipulate the very air she breathes, can be another way of taking back control of her life.

Cedar oil helps bring inspiration to creative work. **Clary** clears the head after too much intellectual stimulation. **Juniper** aids concentration. **Sage** dispels fear and anxiety. **Lily** restores energy. **Lavender** calms. **Patchouli** gets the passions going. **Peppermint** lifts the spirit. **Sandalwood** helps you think in new ways. **Rosewood** quietens the aggressive soul.

They're all natural substances. And they're volatile, so they rapidly disappear into the ether. Catch them fleetingly before they do.

Be careful to buy the real thing. Cheap substitutes, available in many high street chemists and department stores, are often poor quality copies. They'll just get absorbed in your soft furnishings and go rancid.

Useful addresses
Culpeper Ltd, Hadstock Road, Linton, Cambridge CB1 6NJ. Tel: 0223 891196.

CHINESE HERBS

In ancient times in China, a doctor was only paid when the patient was healthy. The logic behind that is unarguably sound, not least because most medicine then concentrates on prevention. Once the patient fell sick, all further medical care was free.

Chinese medicine began over five thousand years ago and one of the many tools in its armoury is the use of herbs. Many Chinese herbs are similar to our own, like mint and liquorice, but then there are exotic things like white peony or thorowax root. The Chinese use anything that grows. They consider dark plums, spring onions and seaweed as herbs. In the West, we're more used to seeing those in our fruit bowls, salad bowls and fish tanks respectively. But as the Chinese have been getting it right for so long, who are we to argue?

In fact, a friend of mine has just come back from a trip to China and brought some novelty gifts back for her mum. Her mother worked for years in the NHS as a specialist pharmacologist, so there's not much you can tell her about drugs, chemicals and medicinal compounds.

For a number of years she's been getting increasingly bad arthritis in her hands and wrists. So her daughter brought back some tiger balm plasters. You just stick a plaster on overnight and take it off in the morning. She came across them while wandering round a local market and thought they'd be a bit of fun. Her mum pooh-poohed them. But the morning after she'd been given them, she phoned her daughter at eight thirty, bubbling with excitement. She'd tried one and had woken up for the first time in years without pain. My friend doesn't want to think too closely about how the manufacturers got hold of the tiger balm, but is just delighted it works.

When treating with herbs, the herbalist will decide whether you have a 'hot' condition or a 'cold' condition. Stomach aches due to too much cold food and drinks will be treated with 'hot' herbs – chillies, garlic, cinnamon, cardamon and ginger, for instance. Mint, burdock fruit, mulberry leaf and chrysanthemum flower are all cold, so are used to treat 'warm' conditions like flu, high temperatures and coughs.

When treating the menopause, the Chinese who tend to look deeper than the presenting symptom concentrate on the liver and the kidneys which they say get congested and deficient at this time. For **liver congestion** you might be prescribed **wild yam**, which is known to contain progesterone-like substances.

Diagnosis is given only after a full medical history is taken. You may have from six to twelve herbs prescribed which you brew up for about thirty minutes at home. The liquid is then drunk like tea.

Herbs have been used by the Chinese to treat the menopause for centuries. You will not be part of an experiment.

Useful addresses
Register of Chinese Herbal Medicine, The Lotus Healing Centre, The London College of Chinese Herbal Medicine, 129 Queen's Crescent, London NW5 4HE. Tel: 071 284 4614.

GETTING TO THE POINT – ACUPUNCTURE

Don't be alarmed. The needles are so fine that all you get is a light tingling sensation. Acupuncture is another Chinese therapy that's been used for thousands of years. And again, the principle is to work on the whole body identifying the channels or meridians that our internal electromagnetic energy moves along. What we would call our nervous system.

Acupuncturists are skilled in listening into this system by taking 'pulses'. In the West, we're used to the pulse from our blood system being monitored to show irregularities. Acupuncturists can pick out *twelve* pulses altogether, stemming from all the organs.

When we're in good health, energy circulates in a continuous flow of harmony around the body. Blocks are caused by bad health and throw up a variety of symptoms. The symptom is a vital indicator of where the block can be located in our internal landscape – the liver, the heart, the lymph gland, the ovary. Loosen the knot, and the energy will flow again unimpeded.

Like many complementary medicines, acupuncture is a form of therapy that uses no drugs, involves little outlay of energy, produces no side-effects, relieves pain and works as an anaesthetic. NHS hospitals are now offering acupuncture as one of their aids in the battle against chronic pain.

The meridians, or channels, along with their energy flows have been mapped out since ancient times. Ancient texts as far back as the twenty-first century BC show detailed networks still used in acupuncture practice today.

The links can be surprising. If there is an internal hiatus, it can show up at any point along the channel affected. A toothache in the upper jaw, for instance, can be traced back to the stomach meridian, because on its long journey around the body, it passes at one point through the upper gums.

Needles may be put in and removed immediately, or left in place for any time up to an hour. Treatment is so closely tied to each person that no two illnesses will get the same treatment. For instance, one menopausal woman's **hot flushes** may be caused by her circulatory system being sluggish, so that will be treated. But another menopausal woman coming in with the same symptom may have **liver congestion**, so the focus would be on her liver.

Acupuncture is particularly good for **mood swings** as its main aim is always to re-balance and harmonise.

Useful addresses
The College of Traditional Chinese Acupuncture, Tao House, Queensway, Royal Leamington Spa, Warwickshire CV31 3LZ. Tel: 0926 422121.

FLOW WITH THE HUNCHES – SHIATSU

Needles and pins may make you shudder. So if acupuncture
is not for you, shiatsu might be instead. It's similar in basics,
but works without needles. There's a subtlety and an intu-
ition to this most gentle of manipulations. It's one of those
therapies where few words need to be spoken. That in itself
can be a relief.

Shiatsu originates from Japan. And translated literally, it
means 'finger pressure'. But the Japanese are an inventive
lot and are just as likely to use thumbs, palms, elbows, and
even knees and feet. Don't be alarmed; it's one of the gentlest
therapies going. As with acupuncture, it works with the
'channels of living magnetic energy', as its practitioners call
the meridians connecting all our vital organs. But they use
mild pressure, and relaxing and stretching techniques to
clear the blocks.

There may be a few initial questions about your lifestyle,
but diagnosis is also done by observation of your posture, skin
tone and also by palpation – a light kneading and sensing of
the muscles. The whole body is worked on.

Shiatsu stimulates the circulation, and for anyone suffering **bloating** attention is given to the lympathic glands,
which helps to clear fluid.

The general effect of shiatsu is to **release toxins** and also
deep-seated **tensions**. After a session you'll feel invigorated
and relaxed.

But something to watch out for with shiatsu, and indeed
many complementary therapies, is that there can be temporary 'healing reactions'. These are a positive, normal sign of a
return to good health. What happens is that as toxins and
negative emotions get released, you may have a headache or
slight flu-like symptoms for about twenty-four hours. This is
good and means your system is clearing itself out. Let it work
its way through.

A session can last for an hour, and you may think it is
worth having a number of them. You stay fully clothed

throughout, but preferably in loose, comfy gear. And you may be sent away at the end with a few exercises to do before the next session.

Useful addresses
The Shiatsu Society, Administrator, 5 Foxcote, Wokingham, Berkshire RG11 3PG. Tel: 0734 730836.

FACE FACTS – FACELIFTS WITHOUT SURGERY

'I don't want lines all over my face.'
'I don't want to end up one of those craggy old wrinklies.'
'I hate it showing so.'

Again and again, I've heard women worried about the fact that menopause ages their skin. Yes, they have dry vaginas which are uncomfortable. Yes, they get hot flushes. But the face caving in is another matter. It's so public. It's so irreversible. And more than anything, it marks them out as 'changed'.

Some women who feel deeply about it choose to go under the knife. Plastic surgeons can, with just a small tuck here and a quick fold there, do wonders.

But it's costly. Recuperation can be time-consuming. And for others there's just something that doesn't feel quite right about allowing a scalpel near the face. In which case, if you do want a facial pick-me-up, 'cosmetic' acupuncture may be just the thing.

Similar to all acupuncture needles, super-fine stainless steel needles, unlike any needle you've ever seen, are used. They are almost as fine as hair and can hardly be felt as they go in. And they're not necessarily put in your face to begin with. They could be inserted anywhere on your body, perhaps your back, your wrists or your big toe.

You might think, your face is being worked on, and it is.

But really it's your skin. All over. And the skin is one entire organ in its own right.

That's because the acupuncturist is again treating the whole you, and there's little point in working on the superficials, the face, if your overall vitality is low. That'll show as quickly as any of the fine lines, loss of skin tone, or muscle texture on the face.

Your acupuncturist will first spend time observing you. Looking at the colour and texture of your skin, the clarity or cloudiness of your eyes, the overall firmness of your muscles and the condition of your tongue. Your posture is noted, how you sit and stand, even the tone of your voice and the depth of your breathing. If you're relaxed, it's likely to be deep. If you're tense, it's likely to be shallow and confined to the top part of your chest cavity.

You might wonder, why all this bother, just for the face? But acupuncture is like all wholistic therapies. It treats the whole person. You may go for a facelift. But your therapist could be quietly working on a number of other areas as well. These may well loosen blocks and tensions, the benefits of which are then reflected in a skin tone that is more alive, and eyes that sparkle.

The main aim when working on skin is to rebalance the hormones. This is not just for menopausal women, but for everyone. And acupuncturists do this by working on the kidney meridian. The kidneys are critical in determining the general level of life force, so they will be worked on, along with the endocrine system, which means a needle in your ear lobe.

The lungs and spleen get treatment as well because the lungs are closely related to the skin. They both breathe, after all. And the spleen affects fluid retention which can influence the rate of skin degeneration. The spleen also affects your body's ability to tighten muscles.

Beware. If the ravages of good whisky and bad men have already left their mark on your face, this treatment can repair, but not rejuvenate. Be realistic. It can firm, smooth and add colour. If you're pretty fit and healthy already, you'll get better results. And it's better to go sooner rather than later.

To begin with a course of ten to twelve sessions is taken over five to six weeks. Then you take a break. Then do one more course. After that, an annual booster may be worthwhile. It costs, but not as much as a surgeon. And unlike surgery, because of the wholistic aspect of acupuncture, you'll come away toned all over.

Useful addresses
Dr Lily Cheung, 15 Porchester Gardens, London W2 4DB. Tel: 071 727 6778.

GETTING TO THE ESSENCE – BACH FLOWER REMEDIES

There's a poetry to this system which will appeal to nature lovers.

It's a quiet form of treatment. And it's one you can do for yourself. It's useful as it encourages a tuning into the inner feelings. Sometimes we can be moving through life so quickly and the outside world can be so demanding that we all but forget we have an inner life. And it's then that the inner life starts to get obstreperous. Moods, volatile emotions and wildly inappropriate negative responses can all be symptoms of an inner garden in need of some nurturing and repair.

The Bach Flower Remedies look at the psychological rather than the physical. In the Thirties, Edward Bach, a doctor turned homeopath, decided that what characterised the illnesses of different people was not so much the many types of physical disease they were all presenting, but the mental state behind them. He identified and isolated a series of attitudes and found that he could treat them with his specially distilled remedies.

The Bach remedies don't use the plant itself, but rather the essential energy found within the flower. On sunny days only, a thin glass bowl is taken and filled with pure water. Enough flowers are picked to cover the surface of the water and then they're left for two to three hours. There are a couple of exceptions, which have to be boiled.

And that's it. The liquid, with its captured essence, is then mixed with a very tiny amount of brandy to preserve it and the result is bottled. Flowers used range from plants like agrimony and crab apple to gentian, gorse, hornbeam, scleranthus, vervain and wild oat.

The claim is that while most medicines treat physical complaints with physical material, Bach Flower Remedies treat the more subtle or underlying psychological cause with this carefully harvested, unseen energy.

We're veering into the land of the fairies here. But bear with it; the system has its own internal logic. A friend of mine never really understood how the remedies worked. But her local chemist stocked them and the particularly enlightened pharmacologist used to advise her. For instance, if her daughter had an exam that day and was anxious and tense, she might prescribe Larch. **Larch** is for those who **lack confidence**. My friend would put a few drops in the girl's orange juice in the morning before school, and often there was a mood change – in the right direction.

Edward Bach identified thirty-eight different attitudes of mind that underlay the thousands of variations of physical sickness, and then broke these down into seven basic categories. Fear. Uncertainty. Insufficient interest in present circumstances. Loneliness. Over-sensitivity to others' ideas and influences. Despondency and despair. Over-care for the welfare of others.

You may hear some bells ringing here. Each of those categories themselves cover a range of emotional states.

Fear can reach from sheer terror, for which you'd take **Rock Rose**, to more specific anxieties, like fear of heights or animals, for which you take **Mimulus**.

Walnut can be good for the menopausal woman. It's a remedy recommended for any period of change that requires adjustment. It's versatile. It helps in the breaking of links. It eases transitions. It can help free you from the past. It's to do with moving forward in life.

Sweet chestnut works on the mind that can see no end in sight, where there is no way out.

Cherry plum is for the days when you feel you're losing control, or going mad.

Olive simply combats **tiredness**.

The remedies come in little bottles with their own dropper attached. You only need a couple of drops for each treatment. Put them in water, or juice, or whatever you're drinking, and sip it over a period of an hour or so. If you're leaving home, put a few drops in a small bottle of water which you can carry around all day.

There's something luxurious and sensuous about sipping a distillation that comes close to being an elixir.

Useful addresses
Bach Flower Remedies Ltd, Mount Vernon, Sotwell, Wallingford, Oxon OX10 OPZ. Tel: 04918 39489.

OOOH! YEEEUCH!

An elixir of an altogether different sort is urine. I bring this story to you in the spirit of true scientific investigation. Research can take you on a path of many merry windings – but this is one that even I haven't tried. I leave you with the thought. You might like to experiment . . .

Rosetta Reitz in her book, *Menopause: A Positive Approach*, tells of a visit she made once to a friend in the country outside New York. The friend wanted to take her to see two neighbours, Josephine and Helen, sisters aged eighty-nine and ninety-four, who were unusually spry and active for their age. The sisters served them delicious carrot cake and mint tea.

The women got talking and Rosetta mentioned the book on the menopause she was writing and her research into hormones. She commented on the older women's good health and liveliness. They ate well, baking their own bread and eating only fresh food.

But they also drank eight ounces of their first urine of the day. And they'd been doing that for the previous twenty years.

When asked why, in some consternation, they said they were 'returning the oestrogen'.

They recommended starting with a teaspoon of urine in an eight-ounce glass of orange juice every morning. Gradually each day you add another teaspoon of urine till all the orange juice is replaced.

Have we come full circle here? After all, pregnant mare's urine is used in the manufacture of oestrogen . . .

Each to their own.

CHAPTER 25

Get feisty –
know what you want
from your doctor and get it

'Is my sex life over?'

That's a fair question to put to your doctor. One of the many symptoms of menopause is a dry vagina and if you do decide to go to your doctor for treatment, it'll probably be on the list of things you want to talk about.

So stick it right up there at the top. It sets the agenda. You are laying it clearly on the line – you don't want any issues ducked, least of all the intimate ones.

If you have a good relationship with your GP, you are halfway there. You may have been going to the same practice for years and feel comfortable, and, most important, confident about the treatment that you're getting. Even so, we know that the average time most GP consultations take is around four and a half to five minutes. You might feel you need more than that. Many practices now run **Well Woman Clinics** which space consultations more widely, giving you more time. So ask to go to one of those instead.

Some women aren't so lucky with their GPs. They're not happy with the relationship in the first place. They don't mind muddling through when dealing with the odd ache or sprain, but it's a different thing when you're menopausal. For a start, the menopause can last a long time, and if you go on HRT, you will be having regular and careful monitoring. You need to feel comfortable about the person doing that.

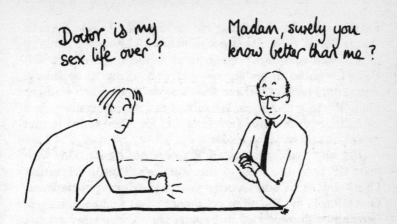

If you are not – then leave. You can re-register within the practice, or leave it altogether. One GP I spoke to was adamant that women should use this option if they weren't happy. She had high standards herself for the communication she had with her patients:

'I need to know that I'm not just programming a woman with a course of treatment,' she said, 'whatever that treatment might be. It is important that we have talked. I feel better if she understands the issues and is making informed choices too. I can't save her poor marriage. Or deal with her grotty job. Or sort out her terrible relationship with her mother. But I can give her the equipment to help her feel better able to deal with those things. I want her to understand what my level of input is limited to. And her choice in the matter.'

There are doctors who are just plain not interested in the menopause. They are not up to date. They don't know the latest, and the complexities of the condition leave them bored. You don't have to be there either.

Or there are the GPs who just miss the mark. One menopausal woman describes going to her elderly GP and trying to tell him how demoralised she was, when intercourse had become impossibly painful.

'Oh dear,' he said, 'that's not very satisfactory for you both.

Particularly your husband! Ho ho. Ha ha.' It was a small thing. But it made her uncomfortable. The doctor actually meant well and didn't mean it to sound quite like it did. Hadn't wanted to embarrass and was trying to be funny. Thankfully he's retired and she's now seeing a much younger man. 'We talk about me. We talk about the menopause. And we talk about my husband. He's just far more tuned in and aware. It's all so much easier.'

One way round the system if you're not comfortable with your GP is to ask to go to the practice's **Family Planning Clinic** instead. Contraception is an issue during menopause. One GP told me she often got menopausal women coming to her Family Planning Clinic because their GPs simply weren't interested. What you're doing is shifting the focus of your initial presenting symptom. You don't need a referral letter as they're 'open' clinics – and once in, you can broaden the scope of your visit.

And there's the **practice nurse** too, who has probably seen it all in her time. She can't prescribe for you. But if you want time to sit and talk things out, these nurses are very knowledgeable and can certainly help sort out any queries or uncertainties, so that when you do see your doctor, you're clearer in your own mind about what you want.

Some health authorities have at least one specialist working in the menopause field who will operate a **menopause clinic** out of the area's main teaching hospital. Ask to be referred there. Clinics can also be found in district general hospitals. There's an advantage in going to menopausal clinics. They're often doing research and so are even more diligent in their monitoring than most.

There are some menopause clinics around the country where you don't need a letter or referral at all. Your local health authority, or local hospital should be able to point you in the right direction.

These clinics are there specifically to deal with the menopause. They will be delighted to see you come through their doors. It gives them work. It keeps their clinic open. You do not have to have chronic symptoms to go there. If you have a poor rapport with your GP, you need a place where communication and understanding are top priorities.

At the back of this book are a number of other alternative advice agencies and centres that can also offer advice and help. And it's worth looking out for local **women's centres**, **women's therapy groups** and **women's health organisations**.

For instance, there's the charity organisation running the **Marie Stopes Clinics**. They are always happy to give a second opinion, without a referral letter from your GP. It's entirely in confidence. They won't inform your GP unless you directly instruct them to. They also have a free advice phone line, if you want some guidance on where to turn next, or if you have a few medical details you want to clarify.

SPEAK UP

The fact that you're reading this book means you're interested in being informed about the issues. Don't hold back about your own views and attitudes. Many doctors these days welcome knowing about their patients' expectations and level of knowledge. This is an equal relationship. It is your body. There are a number of ways the menopause can be treated. If your doctor has a clear idea of what you need and want, you're more likely to get something tailored most closely to your needs.

The very symptoms of the menopause are open to debate. You might find that your doctor responds rapidly to your problem of hot flushes, but the eyes begin to glaze over when you get to your list of worsening PMS symptoms, new levels of irritability and surprising bouts of depression.

You're the one going through it. You know.

Make sure you are with someone who has both sympathy and knowledge. It could make all the difference.

LIST IT

Talking about lists, it may be useful to make one. Yes, some doctors do sigh when that piece of white paper gets pulled out of the bag. But it can save your time and theirs. One of the very aspects of menopause is the loss of memory and lack of concentration some women experience. Better to be clear about your queries than to keep returning to the surgery with vague half-remembered information and general confusions.

Indeed, it can be positively useful to have planned out the visit before. List your symptoms, particularly if they are to do with **irregular periods**. **Times** and **dates** can be so helpful in planning treatment. If you've had irregular bleeding, note its time, and also its **colour**, **consistency** and **duration**. These are all indicators and are useful.

TAKING YOUR HISTORY

Your doctor will probably want to know what medications you're on. Even across-the-counter cold and hay fever medicines can have an effect on you. They're specifically designed to dry out the membranes, and could be the real reason behind something you've identified as menopausal.

The first time you go, they'll probably also want to know something about the following: what form of **contraception** you're on; if you've had your **womb** or **ovaries removed** or operated on; what your **appetite** is like and your general ability to **work** and **exercise**; how you feel in yourself; what your **alcohol** intake is; whether you **urinate** too frequently, and how regular your **bowels** are; if, and how much you **smoke**; whether you've had any major **life changes** recently, like moving, job changes or bereavement. And be prepared to take a trip down memory lane to remember what **illnesses** or **diseases** you've had, and also those of your family, particularly the women.

The tests and examinations you'll probably be given will include **height** and **weight** measurements, especially if there have been any weight changes recently. Your **blood pressure, heart rate and rhythm** will also be checked – along with your **urine** to check for excess sugar, protein or bacteria. **Cholesterol levels** will be measured and there may be a **blood test** too to see if you're anaemic and that your cell count is normal.

IT'S YOUR TURN NOW

After such a whirlwind physical, making a list of your own questions isn't a bad idea either.

Below is a cross-section of some of the things that may be concerning you:

★ How long will the menopause last?
★ Is it hereditary? Will I have a menopause like my mum?
★ What will the hot flushes be like? Are they worse at night, or during the day? Are they physically damaging?
★ If I get one menopausal symptom badly, will I get them all badly? Will I have one or two symptoms, or the whole lot?
★ How can I tell if I'm prone to osteoporosis?
★ If I've had bad periods and bad PMS, does that mean I'm going to have a difficult menopause?
★ Will I get inevitably tired and irritable? Will I have poor sleep, headaches and loss of concentration?
★ What's the best form of contraception during this time?
★ Should I take HRT?
★ What are the risks from HRT?
★ What would be the best dose for me?
★ Am I still fertile when having my monthly bleeds on HRT?
★ How long will I have to stay on HRT?
★ Do the menopausal symptoms come back if you stop taking HRT?
★ What are the likely side-effects?

★ Does it fit in with other medicines I'm taking?
★ Should I avoid certain foods and alcohol?
★ How and when should I take the medicine?

SURGERY

At the same time as being menopausal, you may have other and separate gynaecological problems. Don't ignore them; they may not be part of your menopause, but they should be followed up.

If these problems lead eventually, after all other treatments, to surgery, first of all, you might want a **second opinion**. Talk to another gynaecologist and if there's any objection, find another doctor.

You might find some of the following questions useful.

★ Is there anything we can try before surgery that we haven't considered yet?
★ What exactly will the surgery be doing – removing a growth? Stopping heavy bleeding?
★ What's the likely outcome if I decide not to have the op? Will things get better of their own accord eventually, lessen, or get worse?
★ Is the surgery an exploratory procedure? A repair? A hysterectomy? An oöphorectomy? Is major surgery through the abdominal wall necessary? Can a laser be used instead? Is it possible to do the whole procedure with the least intrusive method through the vagina?
★ What are the risks? What are the side-effects? What are the benefits?
★ How long before I'm back on my feet? How much pain can I expect? When can I get back to work?
★ What will be the long-term positive benefits?
★ Who will do the operation?

Being aware of what's going on around you takes away

anxiety. It's your body. Understand what's being done, and why, and you will feel far more comfortable.

Whatever is being done will be in order to help maintain your health and well-being. If you are part of the decision-making process, the results are likely to be the very best they can be.

CHAPTER 26

Marie's story

I'm the best I've ever been. I've never felt better adjusted psychologically. I've never felt more confident. More attractive. I'm fifty-one. And my periods are still pretty regular. With the occasional hiccup.

And yet it's tempered with the fact of . . . how sad . . . I know youth has gone. I don't think I'm menopausal but there are signs that it's coming. Having been regular as clockwork with my periods, I was suddenly very conscious of the time clock when there have been one or two misses. I'm not the same as I was. I worked for years at the cutting edge of a high-powered communications industry. Then I chose to leave. Now I work in an altruistic organisation trying to change the world.

I look around me at the youngsters. Because it's mainly youngster who work here. They're so sure they know everything. How it should all be done. There's only one right way – theirs. And I sit back and watch them get it right – or make their mistakes. And I know I don't have that energy any more or that single-minded belief in my opinions – but I do have wisdom. They know everything. But I know I have wisdom.

Which doesn't mean it isn't hard to adjust. It's all about how you deal with this thing. I used to be small. I've always been a small lady. Now I'm a large small. I'm quietly watching my body, which I've been casually vain about, slip away. I'm watching the ageing process like an outside observer.

My mother phoned me once years ago. She said, 'It's happened. It's been very quiet. It's past. And I'm still sexy.'

Her menopause was trouble-free. And she's still beautiful. She had hers in her late fifties. I've been and had the bone density check, and done the blood test for oestrogen levels, and everything's coming out normal.

But you have to remember I was a child who took enormous amounts of vitamins. And that was at a time when no one did that. Or they were mad. My mother used to subscribe to the ecological magazine, *Preventions* which was considered more radical than *Marxism Today*. She said years and years ago that DDT was a poison. And this was in the Forties before people knew. We had to scrub all our vegetables before we ate them.

One of my sadnesses now is that I can't run so fast. I was a serious runner. I sprinted for my county and was aiming for the Olympics. I can't cycle or I get bizarre aches. My back gives after a day's gardening, when it never used to. Something is saying, 'Whoops – do we now have you in our clutches?' It's outside of me. I want to keep the kid in me going.

I don't want to go on HRT. I gather you go crazy. I don't want to go crazy. So I'm taking vitamins and Evening Primrose Oil. I don't want the wrinklies.

I have a sense of vanity. I don't want a crocodile neck. I would get a facelift. I'm never going to be a grey-haired old lady. I don't even know what the colour is now, it's been so long since I saw the real thing.

I don't know. I'm beating the odds. My doctor believes strongly in HRT. I'd take a pill. Not the patch. I like to have control. I'm terribly worried about cancer. It runs in the women in my family. But I have all the checks and tests.

The women that I know don't talk about HRT. They talk about clothes and the sales.

Last week I thought I was going – had *gone* crazy. I locked myself out. I never lose my keys. I have two homes in two separate towns and a job in a third. I have to be organised. I got home and there were no keys in my bag.

That is my greatest terror. Over everything, losing my

mind. I felt so vague and disoriented. I got back into a taxi and just sat very still. And spoke very quietly. I thought, if this is that mental disorientation that menopausal women get – there is nothing spookier.

I find anything to do with the loss of mind real scary. I would do anything not to lose that, because that is my worst nightmare.

I have a clarity about my place in the general scheme of things. But I'm conscious of a new physical vulnerability. The one is highly tempered by the other.

I know I'm going on longer than most women. It runs in our family. Each month is an affirmation that I've yet to fully pass into that next twilight. And I like that. I don't want to go there. Not physically.

CHAPTER 27

What next?

The world is never going to be the same again for the menopausal woman. She has been whisked from almost total obscurity to become an object of study for the physician, the clinical chemist, the pharmaceutical industry and the pathologists.

Menopause is on the medical map in a way that it has never been before, as are all aspects of women and fertility. And that's having an impact which we can only barely begin to imagine.

There will be more decisions to make about new and more radical medical procedures than ever before. There will be more changes in the way society shapes and defines the place, and status and potential of the maturing woman. And no doubt that woman herself will probably have a thing or two to say as well.

Recently an Italian gynaecologist had his life threatened should he decide to come to Britain after he implanted an infertile, post-menopausal fifty-eight-year-old British woman with twins.

That story obscured the fact that British fertility clinics have quietly been getting on with the same job and have treated thirteen women over fifty since 1991, two of them successfully becoming pregnant.

Feelings run high about 'tinkering' with nature.

The menopause defines the end of a woman's fertility, whether she's had kids or not. When that fertility is gone, it's possible for a whole new status and role to emerge. This new medical advance turns that on its head.

The figures are so small as to appear insignificant. And we

might wonder what they have to do with the ordinary woman, quietly going through her change as millions of women have before and will again. But it's important because it throws up yet more questions about perceptions of women, and their function, role and 'usefulness'.

It's not the numbers that are important, simply the explosive nature of the principle involved and the precedents set. Even so, that particular advance is small beer compared to some of the discoveries that will emerge from the science laboratories of the twenty-first century.

There have been cases where young women have been fertile, but unable to carry to term, and their mothers have stepped in as surrogates, providing a womb for nine months and effectively giving birth to their own grandchild. Notions of womanhood that have been with us for aeons are being lost in a flash.

On the osteoporosis front, a new form of Vitamin D recently patented in America is being claimed as a new cure. If true, this could put a big question mark over the use of HRT long-term as a guard against the disease.

The new vitamin is called I-Alpha Hydroxy Vitamin D2. It's been developed at the University of Wisconsin and it's thought it could be given to women at risk from the disease in doses ten times larger than those presently thought safe. Once the body has absorbed it, it changes into an active form of calcium-binding Vitamin D. It might stop the loss of that vital vitamin in the first place.

There are suggestions that men may benefit from having their very own HRT. Men's hormone production changes too over the years. It's not as sudden as in women, but they have a form of menopause of their own as their bodies lose responsiveness to their sex hormone, testosterone. Early studies in America are showing that giving men a testosterone boost can re-invigorate those who lose their sex drive in mid-life.

We are moving into a landscape that is going through seismic shifts before our very eyes.

The menopause is a time of physical and psychological adjustment. But a new world is being formed around us even as we make those adjustments. The old certainties about age, fertility and social expectations are becoming blurred. This is not a bad thing.

But it wouldn't be surprising if the menopausal woman, currently coming to terms with her own personal changes, and making adjustments against this shifting backdrop, experiences some confusion. The goalposts are moving. Sometimes it's not exactly clear what game is being played.

We can only welcome any advances that genuinely help to ease this transition time.

As the population shifts and more and more women become post-menopausal, it's an area of medicine that will become increasingly lucrative. We must be careful not to hand over all responsibility to the 'experts'. If we do, we can lose sight of the menopause as a natural process. Let us take what is appropriate and discard what is not. Let us make our own decisions about what is needed at this time, and not succumb to subtle social pressures about how we must, and should, perform.

What goes on during the menopause lays important foundations for the next stage of life. Once the physical symptoms have been dealt with, it can be a time of great celebration.

How often do we long for change? To carve a different niche in life, to move to sunnier climes, a new home, a new job? Whether we act on these impulses or not, they are just outward signs of something inside our souls stretching and growing and changing. They are signs that it is time for the old skin to be shed and a new one exposed.

There is a sense of rebirth that comes with inevitable change. It happens at puberty, with the newly fertile girl-child. It happens at childbirth, with the newly crowned mother. It can happen at menopause with the emergence of the older, wiser woman.

There are many ways to 'manage' the menopause. There are the options of the medical route, or the complementary route, or a customised combination of both. But the only right way is the one that feels comfortable for each individual. However the transition is negotiated, let us hope there is space and time for that new woman to emerge. Because we need those older, wiser women. We really do.

CHAPTER 30

Help organisations

NUTRITION

INSTITUTE OF OPTIMUM NUTRITION
5 Jerdan Place, London SW6 1BE. Tel: 071 385 7984.

SUPER BLUE-GREEN ALGAE
Available through PO Box 10, London N1 3RJ. Tel: 071 241 2183.

WOMEN'S NUTRITIONAL ADVISORY SERVICE
PO Box 268, Lewes, East Sussex BN7 2QN. Tel: 0273 487366.

HEALTH AGENCIES

AGE CONCERN
Astral House, 1268 London Road, SW16 4EJ. Tel: 081 679 8000.

AL-ANON

Family Groups: 61 Great Dover Street, London SE1 4YF. Tel: 071 403 0888.

Baltic Chambers, 50 Wellington Street, Glasgow G2 6HJ. Tel: 041 221 7356.

Room 8, Cathedral Buildings, 64 Donegal Street, Belfast. Tel: 0232 243489.

ALCOHOLICS ANONYMOUS

PO Box 1, Stonebow House, Stonebow, York YO1 2NJ. Tel: 0904 644026.

Baltic Chambers, 50 Wellington Street, Glasgow G2 6HJ. Tel: 041 221 9027.

The Central Office, 152 Lisburn Road, Belfast BT9 6AJ. Tel: 0232 681084.

THE AMARANT TRUST *(agency specialising in advice on HRT and menopause issues)*
80 Lambeth Road, London SE1 7PW. Tel: 071 401 3855.

ASH *(Action on Smoking and Health)*

109 Gloucester Place, London W1H 3PH. Tel: 071 935 3519.

8 Frederick Street, Edinburgh EH2 2HB. Tel: 031 225 4725.

372a Cowbridge Road, Canton, Cardiff CF5 1HF. Tel: 0222 641101.

Ulster Cancer Foundation, 40 Eglantine Avenue, Belfast BT9 6DX. Tel: 0232 663281.

ASSOCIATION OF CHARTERED PHYSIOTHERAPISTS IN OBSTETRICS AND GYNAECOLOGY
14 Bedford Row, London WC1R 4ED. Tel: 071 242 1941.

ASSOCIATION OF CONTINENCE ADVISORS
The Basement, 2 Doughty Street, London WC1N 2PH. Tel: 071 404 6821.

BREASTCARE AND MASTECTOMY ASSOCIATION
15–19 Britten Street, London SW3 3TZ. Tel: 071 867 1103.

BRITISH ASSOCIATION FOR COUNSELLING
1 Regent Place, Rugby, Warwickshire CV21 3PJ. Tel: 0788 578328.

BRITISH ASSOCIATION OF PSYCHOTHERAPISTS
37 Mapesbury Road, London NW2 4HJ. Tel: 081 452 9823.

BROOK ADVISORY CENTRE *(contraception)*

233 Tottenham Court Road, London W1P 9AE. Tel: 071 580 2991/071 323 1522.

2 Lower Gilmore Place, Edinburgh EH3 9NY. Tel: 031 229 3596.

CARE (CANCER AFTER-CARE AND REHABILITATION SOCIETY)
21 Zetland Road, Redland, Bristol BS6 7AH. Tel: 0272 427419.

CAREER COUNSELLING SERVICES
46 Ferry Road, London SW13 9PW. Tel: 081 741 0335.

CAREERS FOR WOMEN
2 Valentine Place, London SE1 8QH. Tel: 071 401 2280.

CARERS NATIONAL ASSOCIATION
29 Chilworth Mews, London W2 3RG. Tel: 071 724 7776.

CHEST, HEART AND STROKE ASSOCIATION

42 Grassmarket, Edinburgh EH1 2JU. Tel: 031 225 5002.

21 Dublin Road, Belfast BT2 7FJ. Tel: 0232 220184.

CONTINENCE FOUNDATION HELPLINE
Dene Centre, Castles Farm Road, Newcastle on Tyne NE3 1PH. Tel: 091 213 0050.

CORONARY PREVENTION GROUP
102 Gloucester Place, London W1H 3DA. Tel: 071 935 2889.

CRUSE – BEREAVEMENT CARE

126 Sheen Road, Richmond, Surrey TW9 1UR. Tel: 081 940 4818.

3 Rutland Square, Edinburgh EH1 2AS. Tel: 031 229 6275.

1st Floor, 50 University Street, Belfast BT7 1FY. Tel: 0232 232695.

EATING DISORDERS ASSOCIATION
Sackville Place, 44–48 Magdalen Street, Norwich NR3 1JE. Tel: 0603 621414.

ENDOMETRIOSIS SOCIETY
245a Coldharbour Lane, London SW9 8RR. Tel: 071 737 0380.

FAMILY PLANNING ASSOCIATION

27–35 Mortimer Street, London W1N 7RJ. Tel: 071 636 7866.

4 Museum Place, Cardiff CF1 3BG. Tel: 0222 342766.

113 University Street, Belfast BT7 1HP. Tel: 0232 325488.

HEALTH AND BEAUTY EXERCISE *(reasonably priced groups nationwide)*
Walter House, The Strand, London WC2. Tel: 071 240 8456.

HEALTH EDUCATION AUTHORITY *(central agency for local community health councils throughout UK)*
Hamilton House, Mabledon Place, London WC1H 9TX. Tel: 071 383 3833.

THE HEALTH EDUCATION BOARD FOR SCOTLAND
Woodburn House, Canaan Lane, Edinburgh EH10 4SG. Tel: 031 447 8044.

HYSTERECTOMY SUPPORT NETWORK
c/o 3 Lynne Close, Green Street Green, Orpington, Kent BR6
6BS. Tel: 081 856 3881.

INSTITUTE OF MARITAL STUDIES
Tavistock Centre, 120 Belsize Lane, London NW3 5BA. Tel:
071 435 7111.

LESBIAN AND GAY SWITCHBOARD
Tel: 071 837 7324 (24-hour info and service).

MARIE STOPES CLINICS *(menopausal advice)*

108 Whitfield Street, London W1P 6BE. Tel: 071 388 0662.

Marie Stopes Centre, 10 Queen Square, Leeds LS2 8AJ. Tel:
0532 440 685.

Marie Stopes Centre, 1 Police Street, Manchester M2 7LQ.
Tel: 061 832 4260.

MIND *(National Association for Mental Health)*

22 Harley Street, London W1N 2ED. Tel: 071 637 0741.

NATIONAL ASSOCIATION FOR THE CHILDLESS
509 Aldridge Road, Great Barr, Birmingham B44 8NA. Tel:
021 344 4414.

NATIONAL ASSOCIATION OF WIDOWS
54–57 Allison Street, Digbeth, Birmingham B5 5TH. Tel: 021
643 8348.

NATIONAL COUNCIL FOR ONE-PARENT FAMILIES *(advice on
housing and social services)*
255 Kentish Town Road, London NW5 2LX. Tel: 071 267
1361.

NATIONAL OSTEOPOROSIS SOCIETY
PO Box 10, Radstock, Bath, Avon BA3 3YB. Tel: 0761 432472.

PRE-RETIREMENT ASSOCIATION OF GREAT BRITAIN AND NORTH-ERN IRELAND
The Nodus Centre, University Campus, Guildford, Surrey GU2 5RX. Tel: 0483 39323/509747/300800 Ext 3396.

RELATE: NATIONAL MARRIAGE GUIDANCE
Herbert Gray College, Little Church Street, Rugby, Warwickshire CV21 3AP. Tel: 0788 573241. Your local telephone book will list your nearest Relate or Marriage Guidance Centre.

SAMARITANS *the name and address of your local branch (open 24 hours) is listed in your local telephone directory or the operator will connect you.*
(Administration only) 10 The Grove, Slough, Berks SL1 1QP. Tel: 0753 532713.

SCOTTISH MARRIAGE GUIDANCE COUNCIL
105 Hanover Street, Edinburgh EH2 1DJ. Tel: 031 225 5006.

SCOTTISH PRE-RETIREMENT COUNCIL
204 Bath Street, Glasgow G2 4HL. Tel: 041 332 9427.

STROKE ASSOCIATION
CHSA House, Whitecross Street, London EC1Y 8JJ. Tel: 071 490 7999.

VEGAN SOCIETY
7 Battle Road, St Leonards-on-Sea, East Sussex TN37 7AA. Tel: 0424 427393.

VEGETARIAN SOCIETY OF THE UK LTD
Parkdale, Dunham Road, Altrincham, Cheshire WA14 4QG.
Tel: 061 928 0793.

WOMEN'S HEALTH CONCERN *(a phone advice service specialising in gynaecological, menopausal and menstrual problems)*
83 Earls Court Road, London W8 6EF. Tel: 071 938 3932.

WOMEN'S HEALTH AND REPRODUCTIVE RIGHTS INFORMATION CENTRE
52 Featherstone Street, London EC1Y 8RT. Tel: 071 251 6332.

WOMEN'S NATIONAL CANCER CONTROL CAMPAIGN
Suna House, 128 Curtain Road, London EC2A 3AR. Tel: 071 613 0771.

WOMEN'S THERAPY CENTRE *(particularly good for eating disorders)*
6–9 Manor Gardens, London N7 6LA. Tel: 071 263 6200.

COMPLEMENTARY AGENCIES

ASSOCIATION OF PHYSICAL AND NATURAL THERAPISTS
93 Parkhurst Road, Horley, Surrey RH6 8EX. Tel: 0293 775467.

THE BRITISH ACUPUNCTURE ASSOCIATION AND REGISTER ACCREDITATION BOARD
179 Gloucester Place, London NW1 6DX. Tel: 071 724 5330.

BRITISH COMPLEMENTARY MEDICINE ASSOCIATION
St Charles Hospital, Exmoor Street, London W10 6DZ. Tel: 081 964 1205.

BRITISH HOMEOPATHIC ASSOCIATION
27a Devonshire Street, London W1N 1RJ. Tel: 071 935 2163.

BRITISH NATUROPATHIC AND OSTEOPATHIC ASSOCIATION
6 Netherhall Gardens, London NW3 5RR. Tel: 071 435 8728.

INSTITUTE OF COMPLEMENTARY MEDICINE
PO Box 194, London SE16 1QZ. Tel: 071 237 5165.

NEAL'S YARD AGENCY FOR PERSONAL DEVELOPMENT
14 Neal's Yard, Covent Garden, London WC2H 9DP. Tel: 071 379 0141.

ELECTROLYSIS

BRITISH ASSOCIATION OF ELECTROLYSISTS
The Secretary, 18 Stokes End, Haddenham, Bucks HP17 8DX. Tel: 0844 290721.

Bibliography

Ultrahealth, Leslie Kenton (Ebury, 1984)

Time Alive, Leslie and Susannah Kenton (Conran Octopus, 1987)

Bone Loading, Ariel Simkin and Judith Ayalon (Prion, 1990)

Menopause 40+: the Best Years of Your Life, Ada Kahn and Linda Hughey Holt (Bloomsbury, 1993)

Menopause Without Medicine, Linda Ojeda (Thorsons, 1993)

A Certain Age, Joanna Goldsworth (Virago, 1993)

Is HRT the Best View, Dr Anne MacGregor (Sheldon Press, 1993)

150 Questions Asked about the Menopause, Ruth Jackobowitz (Hearst Books, 1993)

Menopause, Derek Llewellyn-Jones and Suzanne Abraham (Penguin, 1988)

Menopause: a Positive Approach, Rosetta Reitz (Unwin, 1977)

No Change, Wendy Cooper (Hutchinson, 1975)

Life Change, Dr Barbara Evans (Pan, 1979)

Menopause: a Time for Positive Change, Fairlie, Nelson and Popplestone (Blandford Press, 1987)

The Menopause Manual, W H Utian (MTP Press, 1978)

The Menopause: Coping with Change, Jean Coope (Optima, 1984)

Your Menopause: Prepare Now for a Positive Future, Myra Hunter (Pandora, 1990)

Menopause Naturally, Sadja Greenwood (Volcano Press, 1984)

Overcoming Menopause Naturally, Dr Caroline Shreeve (Arrow, 1986)

Understanding HRT and the Menopause: the Change, with or Without HRT, Dr Robert Wilson (Which Consumer Guides, Hodder and Stoughton, 1993)

HRT: Your Questions Answered, Val Godfree and Malcolm Whitehead (Penguin, 1992)

The MsTaken Body, Jeannette Kupfermann (Paladin, 1979)

The Wise Wound: Menstruation and Everywoman, Shuttle and Redgrove (Paladin, 1986)

The Change, Germaine Greer (Penguin, 1992)

Change of Life: a Psychological Study of Dreams and the Menopause, Ann Mankowitz (Inner City Books, 1984)

Prime Time, Helen Franks (Pan, 1981)

Growing Older, Living Longer, Teresa Hunt (The Bodley Head, 1988)

Ourselves Growing Older, J Shapiro (Fontana, 1989)

The Silent Passage, Gail Sheehy (Random House, 1991)

The Sensual Touch, Dr Glenn Wilson (Macdonald, 1989)

The Hite Report, Shere Hite (Summit, 1976)

Women's Experience of Sex, Sheila Kitzinger (Penguin, 1985)

Scents and Sensuality, Max Lake (Futura, 1991)

Aromantics, Valerie Ann Worwood (Pan, 1987)

The Relate Guide to Sex and Loving Relationships, Sarah Litvinoff (Vermilion, 1992)

Safer Sex: the Guide for Women Today, Diane Richardson (Pandora, 1990)

Overcoming Your Nerves, Tony Lake (Sheldon Press, 1982)

You and Your Adolescent, Laurence Steinberg and Ann Levine (Vermilion, 1992)

Living with a Drinker: How to Change Things, Mary Wilson (Pandora, 1989)

In Our Own Hands, Sheila Ernst and Lucy Goodison (The Women's Press, 1981)

Dealing with Depression, Kathy Naire and Gerrilyn Smith (The Women's Press, 1984)

Depression: the Way Out of Your Prison, Dorothy Rowe (Routledge, 1983)

A Woman in Your Own Right, Anne Dickson (Quartet Books, 1982)

You Just Don't Understand, Deborah Tannen (Virago, 1992)

Raw Energy, Leslie and Susannah Kenton (Century, 1984)

Laurel's Kitchen, Robertson, Flinders and Godfrey (Bantam, 1976)

Guide to Healthy Eating, Health Education Authority leaflet

Living with Stress, Cary Cooper, Rachel Cooper and Lynn Eaker (Penguin, 1988)

Stress and Relaxation, Jane Madders (Optima, 1979)

So You Want to Stop Smoking?, Health Education Council leaflet

Stopping Smoking Made Easier, Martin Raw, Health Education Authority leaflet

Women Under the Influence, Brigid McConville (Grafton, 1991)

Exercise: Why Bother?, Sports Council/Health Education Authority leaflet

Eva Fraser's Facial Workout, Eva Fraser (Penguin, 1991)

What Every Woman Should Know About Her Breasts, Dr Patricia Gilbert (Sheldon Press, 1986)

Contraception: the Facts, Peter Bromwich and Tony Parsons (Oxford Medical Publications, 1984)

What to Do When Someone Dies, (Which Consumer Guides Hodder and Stoughton, 1991)

Bereavement, Colin Murray Parkes (Pelican, 1975)

Everywoman: a Gynaecological Guide for Life, Derek Llewellyn-Jones (Penguin, 1992)

Why Suffer? Periods and Their Problems, Lynda Birke and Katy Gardner (Virago, 1982)

The Experience of Infertility, Naomi Pfeffer and Anne Woollett (Virago, 1983)

Positive Smear, Susan Quillam (Penguin, 1989)

Endometriosis, Suzie Hayman (Penguin, 1991)

In Control: Coping with Incontinence, Penny Mares (Age Concern, 1990)

Thrush, Caroline Clayton (Sheldon Press, 1984)

The New Our Bodies, Ourselves, Boston Women's Health Collective (Penguin, 1989)

Natural Healing for Women, Susan Curtis and Romy Fraser (Pandora, 1991)

An Alternative Health Guide, Brian Inglis and Ruth West (Michael Joseph, 1983)

Experiences in Hysterectomy, Ann Webb (Optima, 1989)

Thyroid Disorders, Dr Rowan Hillson (Optima, 1991)

Coping with Osteoarthritis, Robert Philips (Avery, 1989)

Understanding Osteoporosis: Every Woman's Guide to Preventing Brittle Bones, Wendy Cooper (Arrow, 1990)

Glossary

ADRENAL GLAND
Small glands above the kidney, which control the metabolism and secrete androgens and small amounts of oestrogen and progesterone.

ADRENALIN
A hormone made in the adrenal gland, known as the 'fight or flight' trigger. Produced in response to fear or stress.

AMENORRHOEA
The stopping of menstruation – not due to menopause.

ANDROGENS
Hormones made in the adrenal glands which produce masculine characteristics.

ANGINA
Severe constricting pain usually associated with heart conditions.

ATHEROSCLEROSIS
The furring up of the arteries. Fatty deposits on the artery walls eventually block the flow of blood.

ATROPHIC VAGINA
A thinning of the vaginal wall due to lack of oestrogen.

BARTHOLIN'S GLANDS
Two glands at the entrance of the vagina that respond to sexual arousal by producing lubricating mucus.

BREAKTHROUGH BLEEDING
An artificial period which usually occurs when HRT is taken.

CALCIUM
A mineral essential to create and maintain healthy bones.

CANCER
An abnormal growth of cells that can destroy organs. There are over one hundred types.

CAPILLARIES
Minute blood vessels forming an intermediate system between arteries and veins.

CERVIX
The neck of the womb, opening into the vagina.

CHOLESTEROL
A fatty substance essential to cell membranes, but which can accumulate in the blood, leading to atherosclerosis.

CLITORIS
The female counterpart to the male penis, between labia and vulva.

COLLAGEN
A white substance which forms fibres in the connective tissues, cartilage and bone.

COMPRESSION FRACTURE
A weakened bone which cannot support weight and can break if crushed.

CONCEPTION
The fertilisation of an egg by sperm.

CORONARY ARTERY
The artery that supplies the heart muscle with blood.

CORPUS LUTEUM
A small yellow carapace remaining after the fertilised egg has left the ovary. Produces progesterone.

CORTISOL
A hormone which regulates blood sugar, blood pressure and bone growth.

CYST
A deposit containing liquid or semi-solid matter.

CYSTITIS
Inflammation of the bladder.

D AND C *(Dilation and curettage)*
A common gynaecological operation in which the cervix is opened or stretched (dilation) and the lining of the uterus is scraped away with an instrument called a curette.

DENSITOMETER
A machine for measuring bone density.

DIURETIC
A substance which increases loss of fluid through urine.

EMBRYO
Early stage of fertilised ovum as it develops into a foetus.

ENDOCRINE SYSTEM
The glands which secrete hormones, i.e., the pituitary, thyroid, adrenal and hypothalamus.

ENDOMETRIOSIS
A condition when cells from the uterine wall travel to other parts of the pelvic region and cause pain.

ENDOMETRIUM
The lining of the uterus.

FALLOPIAN TUBES
The tubes which connect the ovaries to the womb, through which the egg travels.

FIBROCYSTIC BREAST DISEASE
A common benign breast condition where cysts develop in breast tissue.

FIBROIDS
Usually benign uterine growths made up of extra muscle wall and fibrous tissue.

FLUID RETENTION
The accumulation of fluid in the body which makes the tissues swell.

FOETUS
The last six months of development of the baby in the womb.

FOLLICLE
An egg-forming cell in the ovaries.

FOLLICLE-STIMULATING HORMONE
A hormone made by the pituitary gland which stimulates maturation of the egg.

FORMICATION
A rare menopausal symptom of a tingling sensation on the surface of the skin.

GALL-BLADDER
This stores bile which digests fat.

GLAND
An organ which produces and secretes hormones.

HORMONE REPLACEMENT THERAPY (HRT)
A combined prescription of oestrogen, progesterone and sometimes an androgen, to replace the hormones no longer produced by the body.

HORMONES
Chemical messengers produced by the glands to influence body function.

HOT FLUSH OR FLASH
A common menopausal symptom – a feeling of intense heat, combined with flushing and often sweating.

HYPERPLASIA
An increase in cell growth.

HYPERTENSION
High blood pressure.

HYPOTHALAMUS
Nerve centre of the brain, working in conjunction with the pituitary to control all reproductive functions.

HYSTERECTOMY
The removal of the uterus by surgery.

IMPLANT
A solid pellet of hormone, usually oestrogen, placed in the body fat under the skin.

LABIA
Part of the female external sex organs.

LAPAROSCOPY
A surgical procedure using a fibreoptic endoscope which is inserted through the umbilicus to examine the uterus, Fallopian tubes and ovaries.

LIBIDO
Sexual desire.

LUTEINISING HORMONE
A hormone which stimulates ovulation.

MAMMOGRAM
An X-ray of the breast, used to check for cancerous growth.

MENOPAUSE
The last menstrual period.

MENSTRUAL CYCLE
A woman's monthly cycle, usually lasting twenty-eight days.

MENSTRUATION
The process by which the uterus sheds its lining.

OESTRADIOL
A natural oestrogen.

OESTRIOL
A natural oestrogen.

OESTROGEN
A group of female sex hormones which determine growth of breasts and start of menstruation.

OESTRONE
A natural oestrogen.

OÖPHORECTOMY
The removal of one or both ovaries.

OSTEOPOROSIS
A bone-thinning disease caused by calcium loss.

OVARIAN CYST
A growth on the ovary.

OVARIES
The female reproductive glands which make eggs, and the hormones oestrogen and progesterone.

OVULATION
The loosening of the mature follicle which then travels to the womb.

OVUM
Unfertilised egg.

PAP SMEAR
A microscopic examination of cells from the cervix to determine its health, and to see if any cell change is occurring.

PELVIC INFLAMMATORY DISEASE
An infection of the reproductive organs.

PELVIS
The bony hip section cradling the abdominal region.

PERI-MENOPAUSE
The years prior to the last period.

PHOSPHATE
A salt of phosphoric acid.

PITUITARY GLAND
Secretes hormones which control many other glands in the body.

POST-MENOPAUSAL
That time of life when the process of reaching the menopause is over.

PREMATURE MENOPAUSE
The failure of the ovaries before the age of thirty-five or forty.

PREMENSTRUAL SYNDROME (PMS)
Physical and psychological symptoms experienced prior to menstruation.

PROGESTERONE
A hormone produced by the corpus luteum.

PROLAPSE
Dropping or protrusion of an organ, usually used in relation to the rectum or uterus.

PUBERTY
The first production of hormones that leads to the development of the reproductive organs.

STRESS INCONTINENCE
The leakage of urine due to loss of tone of the pelvic muscles.

SURGICAL MENOPAUSE
An artificial menopause induced by removal of the ovaries.

TESTOSTERONE
A male hormone produced in men by the testes. Women's ovaries also produce a small amount.

THROMBOSIS
Clotting of the blood within a blood vessel.

THYROID GLAND
A gland in the throat essential for the regulation of the metabolism.

URETHRA
The channel through which urine travels from the bladder to the exterior of the body.

UTERINE BLEEDING
Bleeding from the uterus.

UTERINE PROLAPSE
A loss of muscle tone, causing the uterus to descend into the pelvic cavity.

UTERUS
The womb. A hollow, muscular female organ in which a baby develops.

VAGINA
The birth channel leading from the vulva to the cervix.

VASOMOTOR NERVES
These cause dilation or constriction of the blood vessels.

VULVA
The external female sex organs.

WOMB
The uterus or uterine cavity; a major part of the female sex organs.

Index

Headline Health Kicks

Positive and practical advice to relieve persistent health problems.
Titles available include:

THE PRIME OF YOUR LIFE
Self help during menopause   Pamela Armstrong   £5.99   ☐

STOP COUNTING SHEEP
Self help for insomnia sufferers   Dr Paul Clayton   £5.99   ☐

AM I A MONSTER, OR IS THIS PMS?
Self help for PMS sufferers   Louise Roddon   £5.99   ☐

GET UP AND GO!
Self help for fatigue sufferers   Anne Woodham   £5.99   ☐

You can kick that problem!

All Headline books are available at your local bookshop or newsagent, or can be ordered direct from the publisher. Just tick the titles you want and fill in the form below. Prices and availability subject to change without notice.

Headline Book Publishing Ltd, Cash Sales Department, Bookpoint, 39 Milton Park, Abingdon, OXON, OX14 4TD, UK. If you have a credit card you may order by telephone – 0235 831700.

Please enclose a cheque or postal order made payable to Bookpoint Ltd to the value of the cover price and allow the following for postage and packing:

UK & BFPO: £1.00 for the first book, 50p for the second book and 30p for each additional book ordered up to a maximum charge of £3.00.

OVERSEAS & EIRE: £2.00 for the first book, £1.00 for the second book and 50p for each additional book.

Name..

Address...

....

....

If you would prefer to pay by credit card, please complete:
Please debit my Visa/Access/Diner's Card/American Express (delete as applicable) card no:

☐☐☐☐☐☐☐☐☐☐☐☐☐☐☐☐☐☐

Signature..   Expiry date...................